41 Update in Intensive Care and Emergency Medicine

Edited by J.-L. Vincent

Springer
Berlin
Heidelberg
New York
Hong Kong
London
Milan
Paris
Tokyo

A. Esteban   A. Anzueto   D. J. Cook   (Eds.)

Evidence-Based Management of Patients with Respiratory Failure

With 9 Figures and 18 Tables

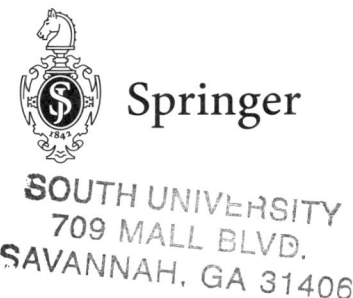

Springer

Series Editor

Prof. Jean-Louis Vincent
Head, Department of Intensive Care
Erasme University Hospital
Route de Lennik 808, 1070 Brussels
Belgium
jlvincen@ulb.ac.be

Volume Editors

Andrés Esteban, M.D, Ph.D.
Chief, Intensive Care Service
Getafe University Hospital
Carretera de Toledo Km 12,500
28905 Getafe, Madrid, Spain

Dr. Antonio Anzueto
Pulmonary/Critical Care Medicine
University of Texas
Health Science Center at San Antonio
7703 Floyd Curl Drive
San Antonio TX 78229-3900, USA

Dr. Deborah J. Cook
Academic Chair, Critical Care
Professor of Medicin & Epidemiology
St. Joseph's Hospital
50 Charlton Avenue East
Hamilton, Ontario L8N 486, Canada

ISSN 0933-6788
ISBN 3-540-20697-3   Springer-Verlag Berlin Heidelberg NewYork

Library of Congress Cataloging-in-Publication Data
Evidence-based management of patients with respiratory failure / A. Esteban, A. Anzueto, D. Cook (eds.). p. ; cm. – (Update in intensive care and emergency medicine, ISSN 0933-6788 ; 41)
   ISBN 3-540-20697-3 (hardcover : alk. paper)
1. Respiratory insufficiency-Treatment. 2. Respiratory insufficiency-Diagnosis. 3. Evidence-based medicine. I. Esteban, A. (Andrés), 1942– II. Anzueto, Antonio. III. Cook, Deborah, 1960– IV. Series. [DNLM: 1. Respiratory Insufficiency-therapy. 2. Evidence-Based Medicine. 3. Respiration, Artificial-utilization. WF 140 E93 2004]

This work is subject to copyright. All rights are reserved, whether the whole or part of the material is concerned, specifically the rights of translation, reprinting, reuse of illustrations, recitation, broadcasting, reproduction on microfilms or in any other way, and storage in data banks. Duplication of this publication or parts thereof is permitted only under the provisions of the German Copyright Law of September 9, 1965, in its current version, and permission for use must always be obtained from Springer-Verlag. Violations are liable for prosecution under the German Copyright Law.

Springer-Verlag Berlin Heidelberg New York
a member of Springer Science+Business Media

springeronline.com

© Springer-Verlag Berlin Heidelberg 2004
Printed in Germany

The use of general descriptive names, registered names, trademarks, etc. in this publication does not imply, even in the absence of a specific statement, that such names are exempt from the relevant protective laws and regulations and therefore free for general use.

Product liability: The publishers cannot guarantee the accuracy of any information about dosage and application contained in this book. In every individual case the user must check such information by consulting the relevant literature.

Typesetting: Satz & Druckservice, 69181 Leimen, Germany
Cover design: design & production GmbH, 69126 Heidelberg, Germany
Printed on acid-free paper   21/3150/ag – 5 4 3 2 1 0

Contents

Evidence-based Management of Patients
with Respiratory Failure: An Introduction 1
   A. Esteban, A. Anzueto, and D.J. Cook

Mechanical Ventilation: Epidemiology and Outcomes 5
   A. Esteban, N. D. Ferguson, and F. Frutos-Vivar

Ventilator Modes:
Which do we use and how should we use them? 15
   F. Frutos-Vivar, N. D. Ferguson, and A. Esteban

Management of Patients with Respiratory Failure 21
   L. Gattinoni, D. Chiumello, and F. Vagginelli

What is the Utility of Monitoring Pulmonary Mechanics
in the Treatment of Patients with Acute Respiratory Failure? . . . 29
   S. Benito, M. Subirana, J. M. García

What are the Best Methods for Weaning Patients
from Mechanical Ventilation? 37
   S. K. Epstein

Venous Thromboembolism in the ICU: What is the Epidemiology
and What are the Consequences? 45
   D. Cook, M. Crowther, and M. Meade

Non-invasive Ventilation: How, When, for Whom,
and What Outcome? 51
   L. Brochard

Pulmonary Recruitment in Acute Lung Injury 67
   L. Blanch, A. Villagra, and J. Lopez-Aguilar

Lung-Protective Ventilation Trials: A Comparison
of Physiologic Effects and Patient-important Outcomes 73
   M. O. Meade, N. Adhikari, and K. E. Burns

Acute Exacerbation of Chronic Obstructive Pulmonary Disease:
What is the Impact of Bronchodilators, Corticosteroids,
and Antibiotics? 79
    A. Anzueto

Ventilator-associated Pneumonia: What are the Accuracies
and the Consequences of Different Diagnostic Methods 99
    A. Torres and S. Ewig

Are the Most Simple Methods Still Useful
in Preventing Respiratory Infections? 109
    E. Girou

Tracheostomy in Patients
with Respiratory Failure Receiving Mechanical Ventilation:
How, When, and for Whom? 121
    C. Apezteguia, F. Ríos, and D. Pezzola

The Use of Sedation and Neuromuscular Blockade:
The Effect on Clinical Outcome 135
    B. De Jonghe, B. Plaud, and H. Outin

Current Clinical Trials in Acute Lung Injury 143
    M. O. Meade, K. E. Burns, and N. Adhikari

Novel Advancements in the Management
and Diagnosis of Acute Respiratory Failure 149
    C. C. dos Santos and A. S. Slutsky

Subject Index 167

List of Contributors

Adhikari N
Departments of Medicine and Critical
Care Medicine
Sunnybrook and Womens College
Health Sciences Centre
2075 Bayview Ave
Toronto
Ontario M5S 1B2
Canada

Anzueto A
Pulmonary/Critical Care Medicine
University of Texas
Health Science Center at San Antonio
7703 Floyd Curl Drive
San Antonio TX 78229-3900
USA

Apezteguía C
Dept of Intensive Care Medicine
Hospital Prof A Posadas
Illia y Marconi
El Palomar 1684
Buenos Aires
Argentina

Benito S
Dept of Emergency Medicine
Hospital de la Santa Crue i Sant Pau
Avgda. San Antoni María Claret 167
08025 Barcelona
Spain

Blanch L
Critical Care Center
Sabadell Hospital
Institut Universitari Parc Tauli
(U.A.B.)
Corporacio Sanitaria Parc Tauli
Parc Tauli s/n
08208 Sabadell
Spain

Brochard L
Dept of Intensive Care
Henri Mondor Hospital
94010 Créteil Cedex
France

Burns KE
Department of Critical Care Medicine
London Health Sciences Centre
London
Ontario
Canada

Chiumello D
Dept of Anesthesia and Intensive Care
Ospedale Maggiore Policlinico-IRCCS
via Francesco Sforza 35
20122 Milan
Italy

Cook DJ
Department of Medicine
St. Josephs Hospital
50 Charlton Avenue East
Hamilton
Ontario L8N 486
Canada

Crowther M
Department of Medicine
St. Josephs Hospital
50 Charlton Avenue East
Hamilton
Ontario L8N 4B6
Canada

De Jonghe B
Dept of Intensive Care
Centre Hospitalier
de Poissy/Saint-Germain
10 rue du Champ-Gaillard
78300 Poissy
France

Dos Santos CC
Dept of Critical Care Medicine
St. Michael's Hospital
30, Bond St., Rm. 4-042,
Toronto
Ontario M5B 1W8
Canada

Epstein SK
Pulmonary and Critical Care Division
New England Medical Center
Box 369
750 Washington St
Boston MA 02111
USA

Esteban A
Dept of Intensive Care
Getafe University Hospital
Carretera de Toledo Km 12,500
28905 Getafe
Madrid
Spain

Ewig S
Dept of Pneumonology
Ruhr University
Universitätsstr. 150
44801 Bochum
Germany

Ferguson ND
Division of Respirology
and Interdepartmental Division
of Critical Care
Department of Medicine
Toronto Western Hospital
399 Bathurst Street
EC2-024
Toronto
Ontario M5T 2S8
Canada

Frutos-Vivar F
Dept of Intensive Care
Getafe University Hospital
Carretera de Toledo Km 12,500
28905 Getafe
Madrid
Spain

García JM
IberoAmerican Cochrane Center
Hospital de la Santa Crue i Sant Pau
Avgda. San Antoni María Claret 167
08025 Barcelona
Spain

Gattinoni L
Dept of Anesthesia and Intensive Care
Ospedale Maggiore Policlinico-IRCCS
via Francesco Sforza 35
20122 Milan
Italy

Girou E
Infection Control Unit
Henri Mondor Hospital
51 avenue du Maréchal De Lattre
de Tassigny
94010 Créteil
France

López-Aguilar J
Critical Care Center
Sabadell Hospital
Institut Universitari Parc Tauli
(U.A.B.)
Corporacio Sanitaria Parc Tauli
Parc Tauli s/n
08208 Sabadell
Spain

Meade MO
Department of Medicine
Room 2C10
McMaster University Medical Center
1200 Main Street West
Hamilton
Ontario L8N 3Z5
Canada

Outin H
Dept of Intensive Care
Centre Hospitalier
de Poissy/Saint-Germain
10 rue du Champ-Gaillard
78300 Poissy
France

Pezzola D
Dept of Intensive Care Medicine
Hospital Prof A Posadas
Illia y Marconi
El Palomar 1684
Buenos Aires
Argentina

Plaud B
Dept of Anesthesiology
Adolphe de Rothschild Foundation
25 rue Manin
75019 Paris
France

Ríos F
Dept of Intensive Care Medicine
Hospital Prof A Posadas
Illia y Marconi
El Palomar 1684
Buenos Aires
Argentina

Slutsky AS
Dept of Critical Care Medicine
St. Michael's Hospital
30, Bond St., Rm. 4-042,
Toronto
Ontario M5B 1W8
Canada

Subirana M
Dept of Epidemiology
and Public Health
Hospital de la Santa Crue i Sant Pau
Avgda. San Antoni María Claret 167
08025 Barcelona
Spain

Torres A
Dept of Pneumonology and Thoracic
Surgery
Hospital Clinic i Provincial
de Barcelona
C/Villaroel 170
08036 Barcelona
Spain

Vagginelli F
Dept of Anesthesia and Intensive Care
Ospedale Maggiore Policlinico-IRCCS
via Francesco Sforza 35
20122 Milan
Italy

Villagra A
Critical Care Center
Sabadell Hospital
Institut Universitari Parc Tauli
(U.A.B.)
Corporacio Sanitaria Parc Tauli
Parc Tauli s/n
08208 Sabadell
Spain

Common Abbreviations

ALI	Acute lung injury
APACHE	Acute physiology and chronic health evaluation
ARDS	Acute respiratory distress syndrome
COPD	Chronic obstructive pulmonary disease
CPAP	Continuous positive airways pressure
FRC	Functional residual capacity
HFOV	High frequency oscillatory ventilation
ICU	Intensive care unit
IMV	Intermittent mandatory ventilation
LIP	Lower inflection point
NAVA	Neurally adjusted ventilatory assist
NIV	Non-invasive ventilation
PEEP	Positive end-expiratory pressure
PSV	Pressure support ventilation
SBT	Spontaneous breathing trial
UIP	Upper inflection point
VILI	Ventilator-induced lung injury
V_T	Tidal volume

Evidence-based Management of Patients with Respiratory Failure: An Introduction

A. Esteban, A. Anzueto, and D. Cook

> *"Success in science is defined as moving from failure to failure with undiminished enthusiasm"*
> Sir Winston Churchill

Respiratory failure is a complex disease process whereby the underlying disease and therapeutic measures interact. The patient's outcome is determined by a variety of factors including how we use therapeutic maneuvers such as mechanical ventilation for prevention of complications, e.g., ventilator-associated pneumonia. In this book, a wide range of topics related to respiratory failure are summarized. The objective of this publication is to critically review and discuss the clinical evidence available for the diagnosis and management of patients with respiratory failure. Presentations in this book are a summary of comprehensive and critical review of the literature with the ultimate objective of improving the clinical outcomes of patients with respiratory failure.

All the chapters in this book have followed a strict methodology for data search and criteria to identify the appropriate publications. The authors searched several bibliographic databases to identify relevant studies, including but not limited to MEDLINE, EMBASE, HEALTHStar, CINAHL, The Cochrane Controlled Trials Registry, and The Cochrane Data Base of Systematic Reviews. Use of EMBASE maximized the possibility of identifying relevant European publications. Other literature sources such as reference lists and personal files were also included.

The target of these reviews was to identify all pertinent information related to adult patients who are mechanically ventilated either via endotracheal tube, tracheostomy, or face mask. Thus invasive and non-invasive ventilation studies were included. We also identified studies that described complications arising from the use of mechanical ventilation which resulted in significant morbidity or mortality. We excluded clinical studies in pediatric and/or neonatal patients. Clinical settings relevant to these reviews were intensive care units (ICUs), intermediate care units, step-down units and post-anesthetic recovery rooms. We excluded studies related to home ventilation and chronic ventilator facilities.

In this book, each chapter describes the specific design of the clinical studies including patient's clinical characteristics, methods, and results. The methodological features related to each topic are also highlighted. The authors classified the studies reviewed using a level of evidence that was based on previous described classifications. The levels of evidence were based on the studies that have an emphasis on preventive and therapeutic interventions. Thus, randomized controlled trials had a higher level than observational studies. However, due to the focus and strict entry criteria of many randomized trials, the authors accepted the premise that observational studies may be better suited than randomized studies to address issues such as prevalence, incidence, risk factors, prognosis, and mechanisms of a disease process. For example, one recent international observational study illustrated how factors present at baseline (e.g., coma), factors related to patient management (e.g., ventilator plateau pressures), and factors that develop during the course of mechanical ventilation (e.g., oxygenation ratio) are all predictive of mortality among patients undergoing mechanical ventilation [1].

The authors used the following evidence grading system:

Level A evidence: randomized trials, systematic reviews, and/or meta-analyses of randomized trials that had a clearly defined methodology, large sample size, and yielded consistent results if more than one trial existed.

Level B evidence: randomized trials, systematic reviews and/or meta-analyses of randomized trials that are of a lower quality, smaller sample size, and yielded inconsistent results if more than one trial existed.

Level C evidence: controlled observational studies, uncontrolled observational studies, utilization reviews, surveys of stated clinical practice, and/or physiological studies.

Level D evidence: clinical judgment, expert opinion or consensus, and/or case reports.

The authors indicate clinical evidence and separate this rating from clinical interpretation. We did not used a quantitative scoring system to assess the validity of the literature search due to the diversity of the objectives, designs, clinical populations, interventions, predictors of outcome and multiple interventions identified. Each chapter also includes 3-5 conclusions that summarize the evidence available, and the authors provide their insight into future research directions.

Several prior publications have focused on critical care to improve our skills at searching and appraising clinical research, including Evidence Based Critical Care Medicine [2], systematic reviews of observational and experimental evidence leading to Evidence Based Guidelines on Weaning from Mechanical Ventilation [3], and numerous workshops and symposia on evidence-based clinical practice at national and international meetings. We hope that this book will highlight the awareness of the extensive and still growing body of literature related to the care of patients with respiratory failure. Furthermore, in the future more practitioners will be aware of the ongoing preventive and therapeutic interventions tested in randomized control trials that will result in an improvement in the management of these patients [4].

Currently, we rely on observational studies such as utilization reviews [5, 6] to evaluate whether the best clinical care that has been determined in randomized trials are actually used in patient management. But, there is a growing body of evidence that this is not the case. There are several examples of the lack of implementation of these studies: In nosocomial pneumonia the lack of utilization of strategies such as semirecumbency bed position [7]; in mechanical ventilation weaning, the lack of use of two hour spontaneous breathing trials to expedite safe weaning [6], and in the acute respiratory distress syndrome (ARDS) the lack of use of low tidal volume ventilation [8]. All these measures have been shown to improve patient outcome. The data suggest that there is a need to develop strategies to change clinician behavior, such as interactive education, frequent reminders, feedback information, and frequent re-evaluation to see if there is an improvement in the application of these measures [9].

In summary, this book on the Evidence Based Management of Patients with Respiratory Failure provides important information to improve patient outcome by clearly identifying the research evidence that we can apply in our clinical practice.

References

1. Esteban A, Anzueto A, Frutos F, et al (2002) Characteristics and outcomes in adult patients receiving mechanical ventilation: A 28 day international Study. JAMA 287:345-355
2. Cook DJ, Sibbald WJ, Vincent JL, Cerra FB, for the Evidence Based Medicine in Critical Care Group (1996) Evidence based critical care medicine: What is it and what can it do for us? Crit Care Med 24: 334-337
3. ACCP-SCCM-AARC Evidence based guidelines task force (2002) Evidence based guidelines for weaning and discontinuation of ventilatory support. Chest 120 (Suppl 6): 375S – 395S
4. Ferreira F, Vincent JL, Brun-Buisson C, Sprung C, Sibbald W, Cook DJ (2001) Doctors perception of the effects of interventions tested in prospective, randomized, controlled, clinical trials: results of a survey of ICU physicians, Intensive Care Med 27:548-554
5. Esteban A, Anzueto A, Alia I, et al (2000) How is mechanical ventilation employed in the intensive care unit ? Am J Respir Crit Care Med 161:1450-1458
6. Soo GW, Park L (2002) Variations in the management of weaning parameters: a survey of respiratory therapist. Chest 121:1947-1955
7. Cook DJ, Meade M, Hand L, McMullin J (2002) Semirecumbency for pneumonia prevention: A developmental model for changing clinical behavior. Crit Care Med 20:1472 – 1427
8. Rubenfeld GD, Caldwell E, Hudson L (2001) Publication of study results dos not increase use of lung protection ventilation in patients with acute lung injury. Am J Respir Crit Care Med 163:A295 (abst)
9. Berc LA, Grilli R, Grimsahw JM (1998) Closing the gap between research and practice: An overview of systematic reviews of interventions to promoter the implementation of research findings. Br Med J 317:465-468

Mechanical Ventilation: Epidemiology and Outcomes

A. Esteban, N. D. Ferguson, and F. Frutos-Vivar

Introduction

Mechanical ventilation with positive pressure is a technique that has been employed in the intensive care unit (ICU) with increasing frequency since its introduction in the mid to late 1960s. Since that time, a number of new ventilator modes have been developed, many of which have been incorporated into routine clinical practice without good evidence of their efficacy or their superiority over other modes of ventilation. Indeed, in most cases physicians must rely only on short physiologic studies performed on animals or small numbers of patients to help them decide which mode or modes of mechanical ventilation they should use for their patients with respiratory failure in the ICU. This situation is in stark contrast to the amount of testing and data required to bring a new pharmaceutical agent to market.

A consensus conference on mechanical ventilation, convened 10 years ago, was unable to make recommendations based on clinical studies [1]. Instead its recommendations were only based on expert opinion, which is of course the lowest level in the ranking of evidence. The conference did, however, highlight the need for clinical studies in a number of areas of mechanical ventilation. In the ensuing 10 years, a number of these important clinical trials have been performed. Two of the main areas that have been explored extensively with randomized trials include: 1) the use of lower tidal volume ventilation to try and reduce ventilator-induced lung injury (VILI) [2–6]; and 2) determining the method that is most effective in liberating patients from the ventilator [7–11]. These randomized trials have been very useful in addressing focused clinical questions, but of course they tell us little about the epidemiology of mechanical ventilation or, how it is actually used in daily practice in an 'average' ICU.

We conducted a search of MedLine, consulted personal files and consulted other experts in the field in order to identify studies that have been published in the last 25 years (1976–2002) that address the epidemiology of mechanical ventilation in a general ICU population. A total of 184 articles were identified. The majority of these papers were studies analyzing only patients with respiratory failure requiring mechanical ventilation secondary to either chronic obstructive pulmonary disease (COPD) or acute respiratory distress syndrome (ARDS). When we limited our search to studies examining an unselected ICU patient population, and which were multicenter in nature with at least 100 patients, we found only four studies[12–15].

The largest of these studies followed, from initiation of mechanical ventilation until hospital discharge, 5183 patients from 20 countries who required mechanical ventilation for greater than 12 hours [14].

Prevalence of Mechanical Ventilation

In one of the first studies that examined the initial results and outcomes following the introduction of mechanical ventilation and the formation of a respiratory care unit, Rogers et al. reported on the 212 patients who were ventilated during the first 5 years in their ICU [16]. These patients had an extremely high mortality rate of 63% [16]. Subsequently, Nunn and colleagues describe a population of 100 ICU patients who required mechanical ventilation, a cohort comprising 23.5% of all patients admitted to their ICU over the relevant time frame [17]. More recently, in the large multicenter population that was used to develop the APACHE III score, 49% of patients received mechanical ventilation[18]. Of note, however, is that this population contained a large number of patients ventilated post-operatively, and among all ventilated patients, the total duration of ventilation was less than 24 hours in 64% of cases [18].

Examining the prevalence data from our three studies, we see that in 48 Spanish ICUs, 46% of ICU patients required mechanical ventilation for more than 24 hours [12]. Similarly, in the one-day point prevalence study involving 4153 patients in 8 countries, 39% of the ICU patients were treated with mechanical ventilation [13]. Finally, of 15,757 patients admitted to the ICU during the International Study of Mechanical Ventilation [14], 5183 (33%) required mechanical ventilation for more than 12 hours.

Demographic Data of Ventilated Patients

In our two recent international studies, the age of patients receiving mechanical ventilation was similar, with medians (inter-quartile range) of 61 (44–71) in 1996 [13] and 63 (48–73) in 1998 [14]. In both cases 25% of the patients were more than 75 years of age. The distribution of gender in both studies was also similar, with men out-numbering women in a ratio of approximately two to one, a finding similar to observations made in populations with sepsis, ARDS, and myocardial infarction.

Mode of Ventilation

Only recently have a few studies become available that allow insights into the way in which ventilator modes are used in daily practice outside the realm of clinical trials. Unfortunately, the number of trials comparing the use of different ventilatory modes and examining important patient-related outcomes such as mortality and duration of ventilation are even fewer.

Venus and coworkers published the results of a survey conducted by mail in the United States [19]. Of the respiratory care departments that responded, 72%

indicated that synchronized intermittent mechanical ventilation (SIMV) was their mode of first choice [19]. Examining actual patient data rather than self-reported practices, and turning again to our three previously identified studies, we find that assist-control mode (also known as volume control mode) was used most commonly in all three studies. Assist-control mode was used in 55% and 47% of the patients in the Spanish study [12] and the international point-prevalence study [13], respectively. SIMV was used in 26% of patients in 1992 [12] and this decreased to 6% in 1996 [13]; however the combination of SIMV and pressure support (PS) was more common in the latter study (25 vs. 8%).

The study performed in 1998 provides additional information regarding the choice of ventilator mode throughout the duration of the patients' ventilation course. Assist control ventilation was again the most frequently employed mode, and in approximately 60% of patients it was used during the entire course of mechanical ventilation [14]. This finding was present in both ARDS and COPD patients alike.

The available information about the use of non-invasive mechanical ventilation, (that given using a mask interface), is contradictory. In a multicenter French study, 35% of the mechanically ventilated patients that they studied received this therapy through non-invasive means [20]. Meanwhile, in the international multicenter mechanical ventilation study, only 4% of patients received non-invasive ventilation [14]. Possible explanations for these different findings include regional practice variations among countries and among different ICUs. Additionally, because the international study only included patients who were ventilated for more than 12 hours, patients who received non-invasive ventilation for shorter periods of time would not have been included in the findings [14].

Ventilator Settings

Traditionally the tidal volume used to ventilate patients admitted to the ICU has been between 10–15 ml/kg. This practice probably stemmed from similar practices which had been used in the operating room, where the objectives are to maintain normal gas exchange and oxygenation and to prevent atelectasis. This method for setting tidal volume is not ideal for patients whose lungs are already injured, such as those with ARDS. Numerous animal studies have been performed in the last 25–30 years which show that certain ventilator strategies may themselves be injurious [21–27].

Recently five randomized controlled trials have been published that compared different tidal volumes and measured mortality as their primary endpoint 10[2–6]. Two of these studies showed a significant reduction in mortality favoring the low tidal volume group [3, 5], while the other three studies found no significant differences between the tested ventilation strategies [2, 4, 6]. Comparison of the size of the actual tidal volumes (in ml/kg) used among the studies is difficult because of differences in the methods for estimating weight. Nevertheless, it appears that the two positive studies achieved the largest separation of tidal volumes between the two groups and may have used larger tidal volumes in the control arms, with or without smaller tidal volumes in the treatment arms, than were used in the three negative studies. Additionally, one of the positive studies [3] deliberately used higher levels of positive end-expiratory pressure (PEEP) than employed in the negative studies, and the other may have generated significantly higher levels of intrinsic PEEP [5, 28].

Each of these five studies utilized a control group treated with a tidal volume and PEEP level that they considered to be conventional at the time that the study was conceived and performed. Given the results outlined above, an important task is to determine exactly what we can consider as conventional during the mid 1990s. Looking only at patients with ARDS, in the 1996 point-prevalence study, the mean tidal volume used was 8.7 ml/kg (standard deviation 2.0) [13], and in the 1998 study it was 8.5 ml/kg (standard deviation 2.0) [14]. Put another way, however, the inter-quartile range of tidal volume in the first week of ARDS was 10.0, meaning that a quarter of the patients were being ventilated with tidal volumes above 10 ml/kg actual body weight [14]. These estimates for mean tidal volumes are similar to findings from the ARDS Network study, where patients were found to have a mean tidal volume of 8.6 ml/kg immediately prior to randomization [29]. Therefore, while we may say that a tidal volume of around 8.5 ml/kg may be termed the most 'conventional' for the mid to late 1990s, it is also important to remember that the weight used to calculate this figure (i.e., actual, ideal, predicted, or dry weight) will influence this number. Additionally, it is necessary to realize that this is a summary statistic and as such does not clearly reflect the fact that many patients were being ventilated with tidal volumes considerably higher (and lower) than the mean value.

In terms of PEEP levels, the two most recent of our observational studies show that the majority of patients receiving mechanical ventilation receive low levels of applied PEEP (=5 cm H_2O), as seen in 78% [13] and 85% [14] of cases. Patients diagnosed with ARDS tend to receive significantly higher PEEP levels than those with COPD (9 ±3 vs. 5±2 cm H_2O; mean ± standard deviation) [14]. Nevertheless, these values in most cases appear to be lower than those recommended to achieve an 'open-lung' approach [3, 30], and it seems that clinicians do not routinely search for so-called optimal PEEP levels.

Outcomes

In our international study of 5183 patients, the median duration of mechanical ventilation was 3 days (inter-quartile range 2–7), and only a small percentage (3%) were ventilated for longer than 3 weeks [14]. When the different pathologies that necessitated the initiation of mechanical ventilation are analyzed, however, we find significant differences in the duration of ventilation. For example, among the 522 patients with COPD, the median duration of ventilation was 4 days (inter-quartile range 2–6), whereas in the 231 ARDS patients it was 6 days (inter-quartile range 3–11; p-value 0.001). Other studies have compared the effects of different indications for ventilation on subsequent ventilation duration. One study found that patients with acute lung injury had a duration of ventilation of 15 days compared to a mean of only 2 days in patients with post-operative respiratory failure [31]. Similarly patients with pneumonia have been reported to have longer durations of ventilation than ventilated patients without pneumonia (11 vs. 3.7 days [32].

The mortality rates among different studies of mechanically ventilated patients vary according to the composition of the groups in observational studies. Additionally one may look at the control groups of clinical trials, but it must be remembered that these patients have satisfied a number of inclusion and exclusion criteria in order to be included in the trial, and as such usually do not represent the typical ICU population. When we analyze observational studies of unselected ventilated ICU patients only a few studies are available. The hospital mortality in one study of 612 patients was 64% [33]. In the Spanish multicenter study, 290 patients died in the ICU, representing 34% of all ventilated patients studied [12]. In a small study of 57 patients undergoing prolonged ventilation, mortality was 44% [34]. Finally, in the international observational study involving 5183 patients in 361 ICUs in 20 countries the ICU mortality among all ventilated patients was 31%, and the in-hospital mortality was documented to be 39% [14].

Conclusion

In conclusion, based largely on three recent observational studies, especially the largest and most recent, we are now in possession of a significant amount of knowledge about who mechanical ventilation is given to, how this technique is employed, and what outcomes are associated with it in a typical medical-surgical ICU.

Approximately one in every 3 patients admitted to the ICU will receive mechanical ventilation for more than 12 hours. These patients will have an indication of acute respiratory failure in two thirds of cases. Assist control ventilation has been found to be most commonly used in a number of studies across different locations, a finding that appears unchanged over the period from 1992 to 1998. The duration of ventilation for most patients is brief (with a median of 3 days), with only a small minority of patients requiring prolonged mechanical ventilation. Finally, the most generalizable mortality rate for an unselected ventilated ICU population appears to be around 31% for mortality in the ICU, and 39% for in-hospital mortality. These data are, of course, subject to change over time as new information regarding the optimal treatment of ventilated patients becomes available, and as existing information is more fully incorporated into usual practice. Future observational studies will be needed to assess for changes in practice over time, to document the 'real-life' efficacy of treatments demonstrated effective in clinical trials, and to review the extent to which effective treatments are adopted into usual clinical practice.

References

1. Slutsky AS (1993) Mechanical ventilation. American College of Chest Physicians' Consensus Conference. Chest 104:1833–1859
2. Stewart TE, Meade MO, Cook DJ, et al (1998) Evaluation of a ventilation strategy to prevent barotrauma in patients at high risk for acute respiratory distress syndrome. Pressure- and Volume-Limited Ventilation Strategy Group. N Engl J Med 338:355–361

3. Amato MB, Barbas CS, Medeiros DM, et al (1998) Effect of a protective-ventilation strategy on mortality in the acute respiratory distress syndrome. N Engl J Med 338:347–354
4. Brower RG, Shanholtz CB, Fessler HE, et al (1999) Prospective, randomized, controlled clinical trial comparing traditional versus reduced tidal volume ventilation in acute respiratory distress syndrome patients. Crit Care Med 27:1492–1498
5. The Acute Respiratory Distress Syndrome Network (2000) Ventilation with lower tidal volumes as compared with traditional tidal volumes for acute lung injury and the acute respiratory distress syndrome. N Engl J Med 342:1301–1308
6. Brochard L, Roudot-Thoraval F, Roupie E, et al (1998) Tidal volume reduction for prevention of ventilator-induced lung injury in acute respiratory distress syndrome. The Multicenter Trail Group on Tidal Volume reduction in ARDS. Am J Respir Crit Care Med 158:1831–1838
7. Esteban A, Frutos F, Tobin MJ, et al (1995) A comparison of four methods of weaning patients from mechanical ventilation. Spanish Lung Failure Collaborative Group. N Engl J Med 332:345–350
8. Esteban A, Alia I, Gordo F, et al (1997) Extubation outcome after spontaneous breathing trials with T-tube or pressure support ventilation. The Spanish Lung Failure Collaborative Group. Am J Respir Crit Care Med 156:459–465
9. Esteban A, Alia I, Tobin MJ, et al (1999) Effect of spontaneous breathing trial duration on outcome of attempts to discontinue mechanical ventilation. Spanish Lung Failure Collaborative Group. Am J Respir Crit Care Med 159:512–518
10. Brochard L, Rauss A, Benito S, et al (1994) Comparison of three methods of gradual withdrawal from ventilatory support during weaning from mechanical ventilation. Am J Respir Crit Care Med 150:896–903
11. Ely EW, Baker AM, Dunagan DP, et al (1996) Effect on the duration of mechanical ventilation of identifying patients capable of breathing spontaneously. N Engl J Med 335:1864–1869
12. Esteban A, Alia I, Ibanez J, Benito S, Tobin MJ (1994) Modes of mechanical ventilation and weaning. A national survey of Spanish hospitals. The Spanish Lung Failure Collaborative Group. Chest 106:1188–1193
13. Esteban A, Anzueto A, Alia I, et al (2000) How is mechanical ventilation employed in the intensive care unit? An international utilization review. Am J Respir Crit Care Med 161:1450–1458
14. Esteban A, Anzueto A, Frutos F, et al (2002) Characteristics and outcomes in adult patients receiving mechanical ventilation: a 28-day international study. JAMA 287:345–355
15. Karason S, Antosen K, Aneman A, for the SSAI ICU-II Study Group (2002) Ventilator Treatment in the Nordic Countries. A Multicenter Study. Acta Anaesthesiol Scand 46:1053–1061
16. Rogers RM, Weiler C, Ruppenthal B (1972) Impact of the respiratory intensive care unit on survival of patients with acute respiratory failure. Chest 62:94–97
17. Nunn JF, Milledge JS, Singaraya J (1979) Survival of patients ventilated in an intensive therapy unit. Br Med J 1:1525–1527
18. Knaus WA, Wagner DP, Draper EA, et al (1991) The APACHE III prognostic system. Risk prediction of hospital mortality for critically ill hospitalized adults. Chest 100:1619–1636
19. Venus B, Smith RA, Mathru M (1997) National survey of methods and criteria used for weaning from mechanical ventilation. Crit Care Med 15:530–533
20. Carlucci A, Richard J, Wysocki M, Lepage E, Brochard L, and the SRLF collaborative group on mechanical ventilation (2001) Noninvasive versus conventional mechanical ventilation. An epidemiological survey. Am J Respir Crit Care Med 163:874–880
21. Webb HH, Tierney DF (1974) Experimental pulmonary edema due to intermittent positive pressure ventilation with high inflation pressures. Protection by positive end-expiratory pressure. Am Rev Respir Dis 110:556–565
22. Tremblay L, Govindarajan A, Veldhuizen R, Slutsky AS (1998) TNFa levels are both time and ventilation strategy dependent in *ex vivo* rat lungs. Am J Respir Crit Care Med 157:A213 (abst)

23. Tremblay L, Valenza F, Ribeiro SP, Li J, Slutsky AS (1997) Injurious ventilatory strategies increase cytokines and c-fos m-RNA expression in an isolated rat lung model. J Clin Invest 99:944–952
24. Muscedere JG, Mullen JB, Gan K, Slutsky AS (1994) Tidal ventilation at low airway pressures can augment lung injury. Am J Respir Crit Care Med 149:1327–1334
25. Dreyfuss D, Soler P, Basset G, Saumon G (1988) High inflation pressure pulmonary edema. Respective effects of high airway pressure, high tidal volume, and positive end-expiratory pressure. Am Rev Respir Dis 137:1159–1164
26. Dreyfuss D, Basset G, Soler P, Saumon G (1985) Intermittent positive-pressure hyperventilation with high inflation pressures produces pulmonary microvascular injury in rats. Am Rev Respir Dis 132:880–884
27. Corbridge TC, Wood LD, Crawford GP, Chudoba MJ, Yanos J, Sznajder JI (1990) Adverse effects of large tidal volume and low PEEP in canine acid aspiration. Am Rev Respir Dis 142:311–315
28. de Durante G, del Turco M, Rustichini L, et al (2002) ARDSNet lower tidal volume ventilatory strategy may generate intrinsic positive end-expiratory pressure in patients with acute respiratory distress syndrome. Am J Respir Crit Care Med 165:1271–1274
29. Thompson BT, Hayden D, Matthay MA, Brower R, Parsons PE (2001) Clinicians' approaches to mechanical ventilation in acute lung injury and ARDS. Chest 120:1622–1627
30. Ranieri VM, Suter PM, Tortorella C, et al (1999) Effect of mechanical ventilation on inflammatory mediators in patients with acute respiratory distress syndrome: a randomized controlled trial. JAMA 282:54–61
31. Troché G, Moine P (1997) Is the duration of mechanical ventilation predictable? Chest 112:745–751
32. Stauffer JL, Fayter NA, Graves B, Cromb M, Lynch JC, Goebel P (1993) Survival following mechanical ventilation for acute respiratory failure in adult men. Chest 104:1222–1229
33. Papadakis MA, Lee KK, Brower WS, el al (1993) Prognosis of mechanically ventilated patients. West J Med 159:659–664
34. Douglas SL, Daly BJ, Brennan PF, Harris S, Nochowitz M, Dyer MA (1997) Outcomes of long-term ventilator patients: a descriptive study. Am J Crit Care 6:99–105

Ventilator Modes:
Which do we use and how should we use them?

F. Frutos-Vivar, N. D. Ferguson, and A. Esteban

Which Modes of Ventilation should be Used?

At the moment, we have a lot of different modes of ventilation available. Unlike other therapies used in the intensive care unit (ICU), such as pharmacological therapies, the incorporation of a new mode of ventilation does not require the demonstration (in a clinical trial) that it is similar or better than previously established modes of ventilation, as long as the ventilator itself is not a completely new device. Synchronized intermittent mandatory ventilation (SIMV), for example, became available on ventilators in 1970, but the first study assessing its efficacy was not until 1973, and similarly pressure support (PS) appeared in 1980 and yet the first publications realted to its use are from 1985.

Search Strategy

A search in the databases MEDLINE, PubMed, and OVID was performed using the key words: [Respiration, artificial/methods OR Positive Pressure Respiration/methods OR Intermittent Positive Pressure Breathing/methods OR Intermittent Positive Pressure Ventilation/methods] AND [Respiratory Insufficiency/ therapy OR Respiratory Distress Syndrome, therapy OR Pulmonary Disease, Chronic obstructive/therapy]. The search was limited to studies performed in human adults, and articles whose focus was either weaning or non-invasive ventilation were excluded because these topics are the subject of another articles in this book. Observational studies, comparative studies, clinical trials, or randomized clinical trials were all allowed as publication types. Finally, the references of the most relevant studies were reviewed in order to detect any important omissions from the results of the search strategy described above.

Results

With the described strategy, 581 articles were identified. Following a manual review of titles and abstracts we selected 82 articles that analyzed the effects of one or more modes of ventilation on either physiological or clinical variables.

A. Physiological variables

In general, the studies that assessed several methods of ventilation compared their effects on blood gases, pulmonary mechanics, or hemodynamics. Most studies examined volume controlled modes versus pressure controlled modes or the effects of conventional ventilation versus high frequency ventilation.

a. Volume controlled vs. pressure controlled ventilation

The arguments for using pressure controlled ventilation (PCV) over volume controlled ventilation (VCV) are the potential decrease in the need for high inspiratory pressures and improvements in gas exchange. Three studies [1–3] in critically ill patients have shown that ventilation with a decelerating inspiratory flow pattern is associated with a significant reduction in the peak inspiratory pressure and in the total inspiratory resistance. In addition, oxygenation was improved in these patients.

One of the theoretical advantages of pressure-limited ventilation may be that flow is adapted to both the patient's demand as well as the mechanical properties of the lung [4]. Kallet et al. [5], in a study of 18 patients with acute lung injury or acute respiratory distress syndrome (ARDS), found that the higher inspiratory peak flow obtained with PCV than with VCV (103.2 l/min. vs. 44 l/min.) produced a decrease in the work of breathing (WOB), so that for an equal level of minute ventilation the WOB with PCV was 0.59 ± 0.42 joules/s. vs. 0.70 ± 0.58 joules/s with VCV. This flow pattern has also been seen to improve gas distribution [6].

Beneficial effects of PCV on oxygenation may arise because the decelerating flow pattern could increase alveolar recruitment. The results of the reported studies are, however, contradictory. Davis et al. [7], in a study including 25 patients with acute lung injury, observed that oxygenation improved when patients were ventilated with decelerating flow (i.e., a pressure controlled ventilation pattern) versus ventilation with constant flow. Further evidence for the importance of the flow pattern comes from Muñoz et al. [8], who did not find differences in oxygenation when they compared VCV using a decelerating flow pattern to PCV. Recently, a randomized controlled trial has been published of 54 consecutive chronic obstructive pulmonary disease (COPD) patients comparing constant, decelerating and sine flow waveforms [9]. The authors found that the most favorable flow pattern for ventilating patients with COPD appeared to be the decelerating waveform because it produced significant reductions of peak inspiratory pressure, mean airway resistance and physiologic dead space ventilation, although with no changes in mean airway pressure and arterial oxygenation. This last finding is similar to reports by several authors [10–15] who compared VCV with constant flow and PCV with decelerated flow. The disagreement between studies regarding oxygenation could be due to the fact that a main determinant of oxygenation and hemodynamics is the mean airway pressure generated rather than the actual mode of ventilation [16].

b. High frequency ventilation vs. conventional ventilation

Most of the studies that have evaluated high frequency ventilation have been performed in neonates and children. The experience in adults has, until recently, been limited to observational studies evaluating safety and efficacy. Most of these were performed in the 1980s and involved high frequency jet ventilation (HFJV).

Hurst et al. [17], in a randomized clinical trial including 100 patients with acute respiratory failure, compared high frequency jet ventilation (HFJV) with conventional ventilation. The therapeutic aim was oxygenation and the ventilation (pH > 7.35, $PaCO_2$ 35–45 mmHg, PaO_2/FiO_2 > 225). Patients in the HFJV group reached the objective requiring a lower mean airway pressure. Recently, a new interest in high frequency oscillatory ventilation (HFOV) has emerged. Fort et al. [18] studied 17 patients with severe ARDS and found that HFOV improved gas exchange and decreased the required FiO_2. Similarly, Mehta et el. [19] found that HFOV improved oxygenation and ventilation in 24 ARDS patients who were failing with conventional ventilation.

RECOMMENDATION: There is insufficient evidence to recommend any one mode of ventilation over another in terms of oxygenation, pulmonary mechanics, or hemodynamics

LEVEL OF EVIDENCE: B (for the specific questions outlined above)

B. Clinical Outcomes: Mortality

a. Volume controlled ventilation vs. Pressure controlled ventilation
Rappaport et al. [2] did not find significant differences in the mortality of 27 patients receiving care in a medical ICU for acute, severe hypoxic respiratory failure (PaO_2/F_IO_2 <150) randomized to VCV (64%) or PCV (56%). The primary endpoint of this study was not mortality, and as such its sample size was far below that required to achieve adequate power to rule out an important difference in mortality. To estimate the effect of these modes of ventilation on mortality, the Spanish Lung Failure Collaborative Group performed a randomized clinical trial [20] involving 79 patients who met criteria of ARDS, randomized into two groups: PCV (n = 42) and VCV (n = 37). Mortality in the PCV group was 51% versus a mortality in the VCV group of 78% (relative risk 0.65, 95% confidence interval: 0.46–0.96). When mortality was adjusted for differences in other variables such as organ dysfunction, however, mode of ventilation was not associated with the mortality.

b. High frequency ventilation vs. conventional ventilation
In the study by Hurst et al. [17] there were no differences in mortality, in length of stay in the ICU, or in the length of stay in the hospital, but again these were not the main objectives of the study. To assess the safety and effectiveness of HFOV in adult patients with ARDS, Derdak et al. [21] randomized 148 patients to HFOV (n=75) or conventional ventilation (n=73). The 30-day mortality rate tended to favour the HFOV group; 37% versus 52% in the conventional arm. This difference was not statistically significant (p=0.10), but again this study was underpowered to show a mortality benefit.

c. **Conventional ventilation vs. low frequency ventilation with extracorporeal removal of CO_2**

Morris et al. [22] randomized 40 patients with severe ARDS who met extracorporeal membrane oxygention (ECMO) entry criteria to one of two groups: 19 patients were ventilated with conventional ventilation with inverse ventilation ratio (PCV-IRV) and 21 patients were ventilated with inverse ventilation ratio (PCV-IRV) and low-frequency positive pressure ventilation with extracorporeal carbon dioxide removal (LFPPV-ECCO$_2$R). Survival of the control group was 42% and survival of the new therapy group was 33% [relative benefit: 0.79 (95% confidence interval: 0.35 to 1.77). The conclusion from this study was that LFPPV-ECCO$_2$R should not be recommended for therapy of ARDS patients.

RECOMMENDATION: There is insufficient evidence to recommend any mode of ventilation over another in terms of mortality or length of ventilation or length of ICU stay.

LEVEL OF EVIDENCE: B (for the specific questions outlined above)

Which Modes of Ventilation are Being Used?

Until recently there was limited data on physician's preferences for different modes of mechanical ventilation. Venus et al. [23] reported the results of an American survey of hospital-based respiratory care departments. Seventy-two percent of the responders indicated that intermittent mandatory ventilation (IMV) was their primary mode of ventilatory support. The main limitation of this study, however, is that it was based upon the expressed preferences of the physicians, rather than observations of their actual practice.

Search Strategy

A search in the databases MEDLINE, PubMed, and OVID was performed using the key words: [Respiration, artificial/utilization OR Positive-Pressure Respiration/utilization]. The search was limited to studies performed with human adults, and again articles about weaning and non-invasive ventilation were excluded because these topics are the focus of other chapters. The references of the most relevant studies were reviewed to detect important omissions from the list generated by the search strategy.

Results

With the described strategy, 51 articles were located. After a manual review of titles and abstracts, four articles were identified that focused on the epidemiology of modes of ventilation.

In the last ten years, our group has published three epidemiological studies [24–26] that reflect the clinical use of each mode of ventilation, as shown in Table 1.

Table 1. Utilization of the modes of ventilation in the epidemiological studies

	1992	1996	1998
	Esteban et al. [24]	Esteban et al. [25]	Esteban et al. [26]
VCV	55%	47%	53%
PCV	1%	–	5%
SIMV	26%	6%	8%
SIMV-PS	8%	25%	15%
PS	8%	15%	4%

VCV: volume controlled; PCV: pressure controlled ventilation;

Table 2. Comparison of the modes of ventilation used in patients with COPD and ARDS (Modified from [26])

	COPD			ARDS		
	Day 1	Day 3	Day 7	Day 1	Day 3	Day 7
VCV	66%	64%	67%	67%	64%	61%
SIMV	5%	3,5%	2%	4%	25	2%
SIMV-PSV	10%	11%	11%	10%	11%	10%
PSV	8%	8,5%	12%	1%	3%	4%
PCV	45%	4%	2%	10%	13%	16%

SIMV: synchronized intermittent mandatory ventilation; *PSV*: pressure support ventilation; *VCV*: volume controlled ventilation; *PCV*: pressure controlled ventilation; *SIMV*: synchronized intermittent mandatory ventilation; *PSV*: pressure support ventilation

In these studies we have found that the most used mode is VCV. This predominance is independent of the reason for initiation of mechanical ventilation (Table 2), and is maintained over the entire course of mechanical ventilation (Fig. 1). However, in a recent one-day point prevalence study, performed in the Nordic countries and including 108 patients, the authors found that the majority of patients (86%) were ventilated, on the day of the study, with pressure-regulated modes [27].

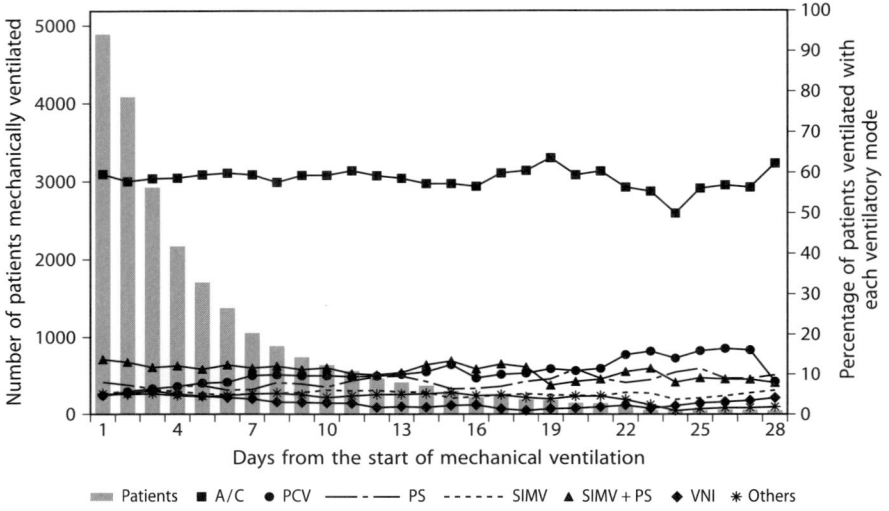

Fig. 1. Daily descriptions of the use of each mode of mechanical ventilation. (Modified from [26]). A/C: assist/control ventilation; PCV: pressure controlled ventilation; PS: pressure support; SIMV: synchronized intermittent mandatory ventilation; NIV: non-invasive ventilation

Conclusion

Our review of the literature indicates that at the present time there is no strong evidence suggesting that one mode of ventilation should be chosen over another. This applies not only to patient-centered outcomes such as mortality, but also to physiologic variables like gas exchange and work of breathing. As outlined above, these recommendations in most cases reflect a lack of high quality studies rather than a well documented equivalence among ventilator modes in terms of effects on outcome. Large, multicenter, observational studies tell us that with this absence of evidence, clinicians are most commonly using VCV at the current time.

References

1. Al-Saady N, Bennett ED (1985) Decelerating inspiratory flow waveform improves lung mechanics and gas exchange in patients on intermittent positive-pressure ventilation. Intensive Care Med 11:68–75
2. Rappaport SH, Shpiner R, Yoshihara G, Wright J, Chang P, Abraham E (1994) Randomized, prospective trial of pressure-limited versus volume-controlled ventilation in severe respiratory failure. Crit Care Med 22:22–32
3. Sydow M, Burchardi H, Ephraim E, Zielmann S, Crozier T (1994) Long-term effects of two different ventilatory modes on oxygenation in acute lung injury. Comparison of airway pressure release ventilation and volume-controlled inverse ratio ventilation. Am J Respir Crit Care Med 149:1550–1556

4. Burke WC, Crooke PS, Marcy TW, Adams AB, Marini JJ (1993) Comparison of mathematical and mechanical models of pressure-controlled ventilation. J Appl Physiol 74:922–933
5. Kallet RH, Campbell AR, Alonso JA, Morabito DJ, Mackersie RC (2000) The effects of pressure control versus volume control assisted ventilation on patient work of breathing in acute lung injury and acute respiratory distress syndrome. Respir Care 45:1085–1096
6. Hubmayr RD, Gay PC, Tayyab M (1987) Respiratory system mechanics in ventilated patients: techniques and indications. Mayo Clin Proc 62:358–368
7. Davis K Jr, Branson RD, Campbell RS, Porembka DT (1996) Comparison of volume control and pressure control ventilation: is flow waveform the difference?. J Trauma 41:808–814
8. Muñoz J, Guerrero JE, Escalante JL, Palomino R, de la Calle B (1993) Pressure-controlled ventilation versus controlled mechanical ventilation with decelerating inspiratory flow. Crit Care Med 21:1143–1148
9. Yang SC, Yang SP (2002) Effects of inspiratory flow waveforms on lung mechanics, gas exchange, and respiratory metabolism in COPD patients during mechanical ventilation. Chest 122:2096–2104
10. Guerin C, Lemasson S, La Cara MF, Fournier G (2002) Physiological effects of constant versus decelerating inflation flow in patients with chronic obstructive pulmonary disease under controlled mechanical ventilation. Intensive Care Med 28:164–169
11. Tejeda M, Boix JH, Alvarez F, Balanza R, Morales M (1997) Comparison of pressure support ventilation and assist-control ventilation in the treatment of respiratory failure. Chest 111:1322–1325
12. Kiehl M, Schiele C, Stenzinger W, Kienast J (1996) Volume-controlled versus biphasic positive airway pressure ventilation in leukopenic patients with severe respiratory failure. Crit Care Med 24:780–784
13. Marcebo J, Vallverdú I, Bak E, et al (1994) Volume-controlled ventilation and pressure-controlled inverse ratio ventilation: a comparison of their effects in ARDS patients. Monaldi Arch Chest Dis 49:201–207
14. Lessard MR, Guerot E, Lorino H, Lemaire F, Brochard L (1994) Effects of pressure-controlled with different I:E ratios versus volume-controlled ventilation on respiratory mechanics, gas exchange, and hemodynamics in patients with adult respiratory distress syndrome. Anesthesiology 80:983–991
15. Merzat A, Graini L, Teboul JL, Lenique F, Richard C (1993) Cardiorespiratory effects of pressure-controlled ventilation with and without inverse ratio in the adult respiratory distress syndrome. Chest 104:871–875
16. Gattinoni L, Marcolin R, Caspani ML, Fumagalli R, Mascheroni D, Pesenti A (1985) Constant mean airway pressure with different patterns of positive pressure breathing during the adult respiratory distress syndrome. Bull Eur Physiopathol Respir 21:275–279
17. Hurst JM, Branson RD, Davis K Jr, Barrette RR, Adams KS (1990) Comparison of conventional mechanical ventilation and high-frequency ventilation. A prospective, randomized trial in patients with respiratory failure. Ann Surg 211:486–491
18. Fort P, Farmer C, Westerman J, et al (1997) High-frequency oscillatory ventilation for adult respiratory distress syndrome—a pilot study. Crit Care Med 25:937–947
19. Mehta S, Lapinsky SE, Hallett DC, et al (2001) Prospective trial of high-frequency oscillation in adults with acute respiratory distress syndrome. Crit Care Med 29:1360–1369
20. Esteban A, Alía I, Gordo F, et al (2000) Prospective randomized trial comparing pressure-controlled ventilation and volume-controlled ventilation in ARDS. For the Spanish Lung Failure Collaborative Group. Chest 117:1690–1696
21. Derdak S, Mehta S, Stewart TE, et al (2002) High-frequency oscillatory ventilation for acute respiratory distress syndrome in adults: A randomized, controlled trial. Am J Respir Crit Care Med 166:801–808
22. Morris AH, Wallace CJ, Menlove RL, et al (1994) Randomized clinical trial of pressure-controlled inverse ratio ventilation and extracorporeal CO_2 removal for adult respiratory distress syndrome. Am J Respir Crit Care Med 149:295–305

23. Venus B, Smith RA, Mathru M (1997) National survey of methods and criteria used for weaning from mechanical ventilation. Crit Care Med 15:530–533
24. Esteban A, Alía I, Ibañez J, Benito S, Tobin MJ and the Spanish Lung Failure Collaborative Group (1994) Modes of mechanical ventilation and weaning. A national survey of Spanish hospitals. Chest 106:1188–1193
25. Esteban A, Anzueto A, Alía I, et al (2000) How is mechanical ventilation employed in the Intensive Care Unit? An international utilization review. Am J Respir Crit Care Med 161:1450–1458
26. Esteban A, Anzueto A, Frutos F, et al (2002) Characteristics and outcomes in adult patients receiving mechanical ventilation. JAMA 287:345–355
27. Karason S, Antosen K, Aneman A for the SSAI ICU-II group (2002) Ventilator treatment in the Nordic countries. A multicenter study. Acta Anaesthesiol scand 46:1053–1061

Management of Patients with Respiratory Failure: An Evidence-based Approach

L. Gattinoni, D. Chiumello, and F. Vagginelli

Introduction

The acute respiratory distress syndrome (ARDS) is an acute diffuse lung inflammation associated with hypoxemia. Mechanical ventilation, despite being a life saving treatment, can cause or increase lung injury. This has been shown in an impressive number of experimental studies both in healthy and in sick lungs [1]. From these data, it is apparent that the lung damage may primarily arise from the use of high tidal volume ventilation, causing overdistension or overstretching of the lung units, or from an inadequate level of positive end-expiratory pressure (PEEP), causing cyclical closing and reopening of the alveoli.

Tidal Volume

Based on expert opinion it was suggested that the airway plateau pressure should be limited between 30–40 cmH_2O or the transpulmonary pressure between 25–30 cmH_2O depending on the lung or chest wall elastance [2].

Three randomized controlled trials evaluated the effect of a deliberate reduction of tidal volume to maintain the plateau pressure below 30 cmH_2O (limiting the alveolar lung stretch injury), compared to a conventional tidal volume [3–5]. In all these trials, the reduction of tidal volume did not reduce the mortality. The ARDS Network trial found, in 860 patients who were randomized to receive a low tidal volume strategy (6 ml/kg) compared to a conventional tidal volume strategy (12 ml/kg), that the mortality was significantly reduced in the low tidal volume group (40 vs 31%) [6]. The positive finding obtained by this randomized controlled trial compared to the other three could be due to many factors, such as the larger sample sizes, the higher differences in the airway pressure between the two groups, and the possible formation of intrinsic PEEP caused by the relatively high respiratory rate used to avoid respiratory acidosis. In a subsequent analysis of the patients that were previously enrolled in the ARDS network trial, it was found that the efficacy of the low tidal volume ventilation strategy in reducing mortality did not differ according to the pathogenic pathway of ARDS (sepsis, pulmonary or extrapulmonary, aspiration, and trauma) [7]. So, from these data, it is now recommended to broadly apply the low tidal volume strategy in ALI/ARDS patients.

However, it is worth remembering that the ARDS network trial just showed that 12 ml/kg is a worse strategy than 6 ml/kg. At the present, the place of intermediate tidal volumes (8–10 ml/kg) is not defined. In fact, for some patients in whom the plateau pressure remains in a safe range using 8–10 ml/kg we do not know of a physiological reason to forego this kind of ventilation, which may allow safer $PaCO_2/pH$ ranges and possibly prevent reabsorption atelectasis due to low V/Q ratios.

Positive End-expiratory Pressure

PEEP has been used, since the first description of ARDS, mainly to improve arterial oxygenation. In recent years, PEEP has been considered not only as a tool to improve gas exchange but also as a means to limit or avoid ventilator-induced lung injury (VILI) according to the "keep the lung open concept". Although the beneficial effects of this strategy have been shown in several experimental settings, we still lack a rational approach for setting the PEEP level in clinical practice [8].

In fact, PEEP may directly and indirectly modify lung mechanics, hemodynamics, and gas exchange; however, the PEEP levels aiming to achieve the 'best' mechanical improvement or the 'best' hemodynamic setting or the 'best' gas exchange do not usually coincide, and we do not know which is the best target.

Increasing PEEP leads possibly to lung recruitment, unfortunately always associated with the overstretching of some lung regions; the final mechanical effect could be an improved, unchanged or decreased compliance, depending on which phenomenon is prevalent (recruitment vs overstretching). The effect of PEEP on lung recruitment depends in part on the underlying pathogenesis of ARDS. Extrapulmonary ARDS usually presents a higher potential for recruitment than pulmonary ARDS, in which consolidation of the lung units prevails over the collapse [9].

Furthermore, PEEP usually decreases, at various degree, the cardiac output [10]. This effect may be negative relative to oxygen transport, but it may be positive on PaO_2 increase. In fact it is known for more than twenty years that the decrease in cardiac output is strongly associated with a decrease of shunt fraction and to an increase in PaO_2, although the mechanisms are still not understood. Indeed, if the aim of PEEP is to increase the PaO_2, this may usually be reached by increasing the PEEP level. However, the PaO_2 increase may be due to recruitment of perfused units, associated with overstretching, or simply due to a cardiac output decrease. Accordingly, we still lack a rational clinical approach for PEEP setting, but, at least, we do know that targeting to the PaO_2 changes or to mechanical changes alone may be misleading. A recent randomized controlled trial compared a strategy with high PEEP/low FiO_2 versus low PEEP/high FiO_2 maintaining the tidal volume constant (i.e., low tidal volume ventilation). The results did not show any difference in outcome. In conclusion, after thirty years of research we are not able to identify the best compromise for PEEP setting at the bedside.

Lung Protective Strategy

The lung protective approach was introduced to limit lung damage by preventing alveolar collapse and overstretching, regardless of arterial carbon dioxide level and to maintain the lung open [11]. The application of the lung protective strategy, with a tidal volume less than 6 ml/kg and high PEEP compared to the conventional strategy, with a tidal volume of 12 ml/kg and low PEEP, significantly improved the survival rate at 28 days (38 vs 71%) [11].

Ranieri et al. randomized 44 ARDS patients to receive a ventilatory strategy with high PEEP and low tidal volume or a conventional strategy with high tidal volume [12]. The conventional strategy group presented higher levels of several types of cytokine in the bronchoalveolar lavage and in the plasma compared to the study group, indicating a higher inflammatory response. Indeed a 'gentle' treatment of the acute lung injury (ALI)/ARDS lung may be recommended, although we still do not know the best combination of tidal volume/PEEP for a given patient.

FiO_2

In healthy subjects, it is known that during general anesthesia ventilation with 100% oxygen may cause alveolar collapse. The most severely hypoxemic ARDS patients are usually ventilated with a high FiO_2 which potentially favor the collapse of the alveolar units with a low ventilation-perfusion ratio due to gas reabsorption. Santos et al. found, in patients with respiratory failure breathing 100% oxygen, an increase in the shunt due to reabsorption atelectasis [13]. However, the deleterious effects of 100% oxygen could be exacerbate by a low level of PEEP which favors alveolar derecruitment. Unfortunately we lack clinical data clearly showing the iatrogenic potential of high inspired FiO_2.

Modes of Ventilation

The most common modes of ventilation in ALI/ARDS patients are the volume cycled and the pressure controlled ventilation (PCV). It was suggested that the decelerating flow of the PCV may ameliorate the gas exchange compared to the constant flow of volume cycled ventilation. However, at present, no relevant differences between volume cycled ventilation and PCV have been reported relative to gas exchange, hemodynamics, or lung mechanic [14].

Prone Position

The prone position is used to improve the arterial oxygenation in ALI/ARDS patients. The rate of response is around 60–70 %. At present, it is not possible to predict which patients can favorably respond to the prone position.

There is only one multicenter study that evaluated the effect of prone position on the outcome [15]. In this randomized trial, 304 patients were enrolled and randomized to a predefined prone position strategy (i.e., at least 6 hours daily for ten days) and to a conventional strategy (i.e., supine). The mortality did not significantly differ between the prone and the supine group at the end of day 10 (21 vs 25 %), at the time of discharge from intensive care (51 vs 48 %), or at 6 months (62 vs 59 %). However, these negative results could be explained by the inadequate statistical power, the short length of the prone position (i.e., an average of only 7 hours per day), and the limitation of the prone position to only 10 days.

In a post hoc analysis, a significantly lower 10 day mortality was found in the prone group compared to the supine group in the patients with the lowest PaO_2/FiO_2 (< 88 mmHg), with the highest Simplified Acute Physiology Score (SAPS > 49) and the highest tidal volume (> 12 ml/Kg).

At present, the prone position still remains a rescue life saving maneuver in severe hypoxemia. Its place in the clinical prevention of lung damage and outcome is still not defined.

Recruitment Maneuver/derecruitment

The American Consensus Conference on ARDS suggested the periodic use of recruiting maneuvers to prevent lung atelectasis during low tidal volume ventilation [2]. To recruit the lung is mandatory to provide a sufficient opening pressure, i.e., transpulmonary pressure, which may be as high as 35–40 cmH$_2$O. Targeting the recruitment maneuver to the predetermined airway pressure may be inappropriate in patients with increased chest wall elastance/increased abdominal pressure. In fact, for a given applied airway pressure, the resulting transpulmonary pressure depends on the relationship between chest wall and total elastance of the respiratory system. Accordingly Grasso et al. recently demonstrated in 22 ARDS patients that the application of a recruitment maneuver (i.e., continuous positive airway pressure [CPAP] of 40 cmH$_2$O for 40 seconds) was effective in improving arterial oxygenation only in patients with early ARDS (average time spent on mechanical ventilation 1 day) [16]. This could be explained by the higher transpulmonary pressure (29 vs 18 cmH$_2$O) that was reached in responders compared to nonresponders. The nonresponders presented with a stiffer chest wall. Interestingly, in the nonresponders, recruitment maneuvers caused a significant decrease in arterial pressure and cardiac output that returned to baseline values after the recruitment maneuver.

We found in 10 ARDS patients, that a recruitment maneuver (performed as periodic increases of plateau pressure to 45 cmH$_2$O) significantly increased the arterial oxygenation from 93 to 138 mmHg and the end expiratory lung volume from 1.5 to 1.9 l [17]. When considering the pathogenesis of ARDS, the recruitment maneuver was more effective in extrapulmonary than in pulmonary ARDS.

Once opened, the recruited lung must be kept open over time. Physiologically it is well known that what causes the derecruitment is eihter a progressive appearance of reabsorption atelectasis due to a low V/Q ratio in some lung regions or a PEEP level inadequate to prevent the compression atelectasis. Interestingly, Richard et

Table 1. Levels of evidence for the current studies in ARDS/ALI

		Evidence
Tidal volume	Brochard et al. [3]	B
	Stewart et al. [4]	B
	Brower et al. [5]	B
	ARDS Network. [6]	B
PEEP	Dreyfuss et al. [1]	C
	Gattinoni et al. [9]	C
	Dantzker et al. [10]	C
Lung Protective Strategy	Amato et al. [11]	B
	Ranieri et al. [12]	B
FiO_2	Santos et al. [13]	C
Prone position	Artigas et al. [2]	D
	Gattinoni et al. [15]	B
Recruitment maneuvers	Artigas et al. [2]	D
	Grasso et al. [16]	C
	Pelosi et al. [17]	C
	Lapinsky et al. [19]	C

al. demonstrated that a reduction of tidal volume from 10 to 6 ml/kg caused significant alveolar derecruitment [18]. This may be due to a low alveolar ventilation with high inspired high FiO_2 and hypercapnia. In these conditions, the effects of recruitment maneuvers are rapidly lost because of reabsorption atelectasis. The maintenance of the recruitment effect on gas exchange also depends on the adequacy of PEEP levels. It has been shown that oxygenation is usually maintained by increasing PEEP (may last up to four hours if the PEEP level is adequate) [19] and may be rapidly lost if the PEEP is inadequate.

Indeed the recruitment maneuver cannot be rationalized without considering the derecruitment as the two phenomena are deeply related. Accordingly, Villagra et al. showed that a recruitment maneuver in ARDS patients ventilated with the lung protective strategy was ineffective in improving the arterial oxygenation in the majority of the patients [18]. Probably the lung was already fully recruited by the high level of PEEP used in these patients and the majority of them had pulmonary ARDS with less potential for recruitment compared to extrapulmonary ARDS. In summary, before using a recruitment maneuver we should consider:
- the potential for recruitment in a given patient
- the transpulmonary pressure to which the recruitment maneuver must be targeted
- the airway pressure which must be applied to reach the targeted transpulmonary pressure
- the ventilatory setting (PEEP and alveolar ventilation) to be used after recruitment to maintain the recruitment effects.

Unfortunately the method, the duration, and the timing of recruitment maneuvers are still not defined. We must also consider the possible negative effects of recrutiment maneuvers in reducing cardiac output and arterial pressure and in inducing barotrauma.

References

1. Dreyfuss D, Saumon G (1998) Ventilator-induced lung injury: lessons from experimental studies. Am J Respir Crit Care Med 157:294–323
2. Artigas A, Bernard GR, Carlet J, et al (1998) The American-European Consensus Conference on ARDS, part 2: Ventilatory, pharmacologic, supportive therapy, study design strategies, and issues related to recovery and remodeling. Acute respiratory distress syndrome. Am J Respir Crit Care Med 157:1332–1347
3. Brochard L, Roudot-Thoraval F, Roupie E, et al (1998) Tidal volume reduction for prevention of ventilator-induced lung injury in acute respiratory distress syndrome. The Multicenter Trail Group on Tidal Volume reduction in ARDS. Am J Respir Crit Care Med 158:1831–1838
4. Stewart TE, Meade MO, Cook DJ, et al (1998) Evaluation of a ventilation strategy to prevent barotrauma in patients at high risk for acute respiratory distress syndrome. Pressure- and Volume-Limited Ventilation Strategy Group. N Engl J Med 338:355–361
5. Brower RG, Shanholtz CB, Fessler HE, et al (1999) Prospective, randomized, controlled clinical trial comparing traditional versus reduced tidal volume ventilation in acute respiratory distress syndrome patients. Crit Care Med 27:1492–1498
6. The Acute Respiratory Distress Syndrome Network (2000) Ventilation with lower tidal volumes as compared with traditional tidal volumes for acute lung injury and the acute respiratory distress syndrome. N Engl J Med 342:1301–1308
7. Eisner MD, Thompson T, Hudson LD, et al (2001) Efficacy of low tidal volume ventilation in patients with different clinical risk factors for acute lung injury and the acute respiratory distress syndrome. Am J Respir Crit Care Med 164:231–236
8. Dreyfuss D, Saumon G (2002) Evidence-based medicine or fuzzy logic: what is best for ARDS management? Intensive Care Med 28:230–234
9. Gattinoni L, Pelosi P, Suter PM, Pedoto A, Vercesi P, Lissoni A (1998) Acute respiratory distress syndrome caused by pulmonary and extrapulmonary disease. Different syndromes? Am J Respir Crit Care Med 158:3–11
10. Dantzker DR, Lynch JP, Weg JG (1980) Depression of cardiac output is a mechanism of shunt reduction in the therapy of acute respiratory failure. Chest 77:636–642
11. Amato MB, Barbas CS, Medeiros DM, et al (1998) Effect of a protective-ventilation strategy on mortality in the acute respiratory distress syndrome. N Engl J Med 338:347–354
12. Ranieri VM, Suter PM, Tortorella C, et al (1999) Effect of mechanical ventilation on inflammatory mediators in patients with acute respiratory distress syndrome: a randomized controlled trial. JAMA 282:54–61
13. Santos C, Ferrer M, Roca J, Torres A, Hernandez C, Rodriguez-Roisin R (2000) Pulmonary gas exchange response to oxygen breathing in acute lung injury. Am J Respir Crit Care Med 161:26–31
14. Lessard MR, Guerot E, Lorino H, Lemaire F, Brochard L (1994) Effects of pressure-controlled with different I:E ratios versus volume-controlled ventilation on respiratory mechanics, gas exchange, and hemodynamics in patients with adult respiratory distress syndrome. Anesthesiology 80:983–991
15. Gattinoni L, Tognoni G, Pesenti A, et al (2001) Effect of prone positioning on the survival of patients with acute respiratory failure. N Engl J Med 345:568–573

16. Grasso S, Mascia L, Del Turco M, et al (2002) Effects of recruiting maneuvers in patients with acute respiratory distress syndrome ventilated with protective ventilatory strategy. Anesthesiology 96:795–802
17. Pelosi P, Cadringher P, Bottino N, et al (1999) Sigh in acute respiratory distress syndrome. Am J Respir Crit Care Med 159:872–880
18. Richard JC, Maggiore SM, Jonson B, Mancebo J, Lemaire F, Brochard L (2001) Influence of tidal volume on alveolar recruitment. Respective role of PEEP and a recruitment maneuver. Am J Respir Crit Care Med 163:1609–1613
19. Lapinsky SE, Aubin M, Mehta S, Boiteau P, Slutsky AS (1999) Safety and efficacy of a sustained inflation for alveolar recruitment in adults with respiratory failure. Intensive Care Med 25:1297–1301

What is the Utility of Monitoring Pulmonary Mechanics in the Treatment of Patients with Acute Respiratory Failure?

S. Benito, M. Subirana, J. M. García

Introduction

Monitoring is to use an instrument with the purpose of making a measurement, rather than of providing treatment. The variable measured can be of interest from a physiopathologic point of view, for later adjustment, or it may be associated with patient outcome. In either case, the adjustment of the variables should be to the patient's benefit.

Pulmonary mechanics is the method of physiological measures used for diagnostic purposes and which allows exploration of the mechanical properties of the total respiratory system. It can be adapted to patients under mechanical ventilation, as they can be easily sedated in order to obtain the measurement. Reduced to the simplicity of a loop, it provides information about the complexity of the thoracic system: the lung, airways, ribcage, respiratory muscles, and abdomen. Pulmonary mechanics analyses the respiratory movement; the components involved are described in the equation of the movement, these being the elastic properties, the resistance to flow, and inertia. For clinical study, inertia can be ruled out. Pulmonary parenchyma is responsible for the elastic behaviour and the airway is responsible for airflow resistance. In order to eliminate the non-elastic forces, the exploration must be performed under static conditions.

Evidence-based medicine (EBM) methodology has been extensively developed in recent years, and applied to the evaluation of diagnostic tests. In this chapter on the utility of pulmonary mechanics monitoring, the EBM strategy has been used and results are commented on.

Study Identification

The databases MEDLINE, CINAHL, and the Cochrane Library were consulted by means of a structured electronic search. A total of 255 article summaries and four systematic reviews were obtained. Once the relevant abstracts were read, the originals were recovered and, from their bibliography, additional articles were obtained. For this chapter, 64 original articles were analyzed, covering a period of thirty years.

Evaluation of Diagnostic Examination Studies

According to the EBM criteria (Table 1) for critical appraisal, diagnostic studies must be compared with a standard reference and in the population of patients that will be later used in clinical practice. The studies must provide the rates of probability of the examination results or the necessary data for their calculation. They should be reproducible and useful for patient management and contribute to modification of treatment. The degree of recommendation and the levels of evidence for the diagnostic examinations differ depending on the topic in question. Systematic reviews prioritize cohort studies that validate the quality of the test and are of high specificity.

Critical appraisal of the 64 retrieved articles shows they do not meet the EBM criteria and should be rejected. To analyze diagnostic tests based on clinical studies and final outcomes, EBM is possibly a very well consolidated methodology but it is less useful in evaluating results from basic research and physiopathology which includes pulmonary mechanics studies.

Table 1. Oxford Centre for Evidence-based Medicine Levels of Evidence for Diagnosis (May 2001), adapted from http://www.cebm.net/levels_of_evidence.asp#levels

Level	
1a	SR (with homogeneity) of Level 1 diagnostic studies; CDR* with 1b studies from different clinical centres
1b	Validating cohort study with good reference standards; or CRD* tested within one clinical centre
1c	Absolute SpPins and SnNouts
2a	SR (with homogeneity) of Level >2 diagnostic studies
2b	Exploratory cohort study with good reference standards; CDR* after derivation, or validated only on split-sample** or databases
3a	SR (with homogeneity) of 3b and better studies
3b	Non-consecutive study; or without consistently applied reference standards
4	Case-control study, poor or non-independent reference standard
5	Expert opinion without explicit critical appraisal, or based on physiology, bench research or "first principles"

SR: systematic review; *: Clinical Decision Rule -These are algorithms or scoring systems which lead to a prognostic estimation or a diagnostic category. $ An "Absolute SpPin" is a diagnostic finding whose Specificity is so high that a Positive result rules-in the diagnosis. An "Absolute SnNout" is a diagnostic finding whose Sensitivity is so high that a Negative result rules-out the diagnosis. ** Split-sample validation is achieved by collecting all the information in a single tranche, then artificially dividing this into "derivation" and "validation" samples.

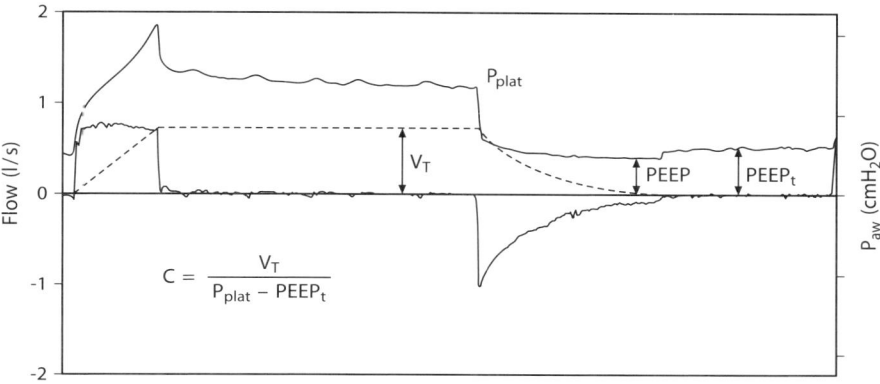

Fig. 1. Total compliance of the respiratory system during mechanical ventilation

Analysis of Intervention: Compliance

How is it Measured?

1. **Total compliance of the respiratory system:** We obtain the value of the compliance by dividing the tidal volume by the total positive end-expiratory pressure (PEEP, which includes intrinsic PEEP) subtracted from the pressure measurement at zero flow with a pause of 1.2 sec at the end of inspiration (Fig 1). The compliance value depends on the value of the increase in induced volume and the pulmonary volume, specifically of the functional residual capacity (FRC) and the increase produced by the PEEP applied [1].
2. **Pressure-Volume (P/V) loop:** The patient should be supine, sedated, and paralyzed. After suctioning the secretions and producing a deep insufflation the patient is connected to a syringe of 2 l and to a pressure transducer, while the volume is set at FRC. 100 millilitres are insufflated; after a pause of 1 second, another 100 millilitres are insufflated, until reaching 25 ml/kg or 40 cmH_2O of airway pressure (Paw). Deflection follows this point and is performed with the same pauses and decrements. The pause points are joined [2].

What Information does it Give?

The P/V loop yields the lower inflection point (LIP) and upper inflection point (UIP), the compliance in various portions of the loop, and hysteresis. The pulmonary distensibility status from FRC to total lung volume (TLV), can be explored by means of the P/V loop in its static condition, by tidal volume loops at different PEEP increases, and by an airway pressure curve at the same tidal volume value and increses of PEEP values (Fig. 2).

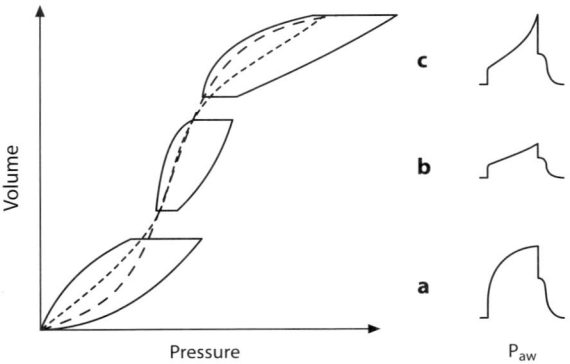

Fig 2. P/V loop and, at different PEEP increases, tidal volume loops and airway pressure curves.

Is it the Only Way to obtain these Data?

In addition to the supersyringe system [1], systems of continuous flow and occlusion have been described [3, 4].

What are the risks of the measurement?

Performing a P/V loop technique is well tolerated, although it can cause changes in oxygenation and hemodynamics. For this reason, patients must be strictly monitored during the maneuver [5].

Utility of Measurement of Pulmonary Mechanics

Is the P/V Loop Measurement Effective in Patients with Acute Respiratory Failure?

Models of the P/V loop have been described to correspond with the thorax X-ray in patients with different stages of acute respiratory distress syndrome (ARDS) [2]. The behaviour of the P/V loop has been related to the amount of healthy lung and the recruitment of pulmonary zones when using varying values of PEEP [6, 7], as well as to the pulmonary or extrapulmonary origin of the ARDS [8].

Is the Compliance Measurement in Patients with Acute Respiratory Failure Effective in Deciding the Value of PEEP to set on the Ventilator?

Table 2 shows articles that used the inflection pressure as a value to decide the level of PEEP in mechanically ventilated patients. Note that for some authors, LIP is the value of PEEP to improve oxygenation [2] and ventilation [9]. Others

Table 2. PEEP versus LIP

Study	Design	Pathology	N°	Technique	Result
Matamis [2]	Cross-sectional	ARDS	19	Syringe	LIP = PEEP
Gattinoni [6]	Cross-sectional	ARF	20	Syringe	Best PEEP> LIP most of the recruitment
Blanch [9]	Cross-sectional	ARF	13	Syringe	LIP= PEEP = ↓ (PaCo2-PetCO2)
Brunet [10]	Cross-sectional	ARDS	8	Syringe	PEEP = blood gases; optimized P-Vc
Jonson [11]	Cross-sectional	ALI	11	Computer-controlled ventilator	Recruitment occurs far above LIP
Richard [12]	Cross-sectional	ALI	15	Computer-controlled ventilator	PEEP = or above LIP → alveolar instability
Maggiore [13]	Cross-sectional	ALI	16	Computer-controlled ventilator	LIP is a poor predictor of alveolar Closure
Mancini [14]	Cross-sectional	ARDS	8	Syringe	P flex + 2 ↑ oxygenation (PVS)
Amato [15]	Randomized	ARDS	53	Insp. Static P/V curve	PEEP= LIP+2; protective ventilation ↓ mortality

ARDS: acute respiratory dictress syndrome; *ARF*: acute respiratory failure; *ALI*: acute lung injury; *LIP*: lower inflection point; *PEEP*: positive end-expiratory pressure; *P/V*: pressure/volume

recommend setting the level of PEEP to improve arterial blood gases and only in some cases with the loop [10]; still other authors recommend the use of discretely superior values [6, 14, 15]. For others recruitment that is tried with PEEP cannot be assured with PEEP levels equal to the LIP [11–13]. The work of Amato and colleagues [15] deserves a separate analysis. It was a randomized controlled trial, with a ventilatory technique of lung protection in which it used a value of PEEP calculated from the P/V loop. With this modality a mortality reduction in relation to the control group was observed.

Is the Measurement of Compliance Effective in Diminishing the Pulmonary Injury induced by the Ventilator in Patients with Acute Respiratory Failure?

Richard et al. [12] analyzed the risk of alveolar derecruitment with low tidal volumes when the pulmonary protection modality is used. They concluded that to avoid derecruitment, a PEEP level equal to LIP +4 can be used, or periodic recruitment maneuvers can be made. Takeuchi et al. [16] analyzed the most appropriate method to determine PEEP during the ventilatory strategy of lung protection. Although an experimental model is not applicable for an EBM review, the conclusions may be worthy of consideration for this question. PEEP calculated on the basis of the P/V loop diminished pulmonary injury as compared with the PEEP calculated by the suitable oxygenation method, and the 2 cmH$_2$O below the LIP was more effective.

Conclusion

- The P/V loop provides information about the state of the lung in the ARDS, and has helped to improve our understanding of the lung in mechanical ventilation.
- The most adequate area to ventilate the patient is possibly between the LIP and the UIP. This would suggest using the PEEP and the tidal volume placed outside the zones of derecruitment and overdistension.
- In its present state, the technique cannot be recommended for general use. In addition, due to a lack of suitable studies, its clinical implications are not well known.

Future investigation

- Systems to perform a P/V loop with continuous flow by means of the ventilator.
- Standardization of the maneuver. Previous history of volume (insufflation, opening maneuver) in zero end-expiratory pressure (ZEEP), insufflation to 40 cmH$_2$O, deflation.
- Help with ventilation decision-making (tidal volume, PEEP). Comparative studies in homogenous patients (LIP, +2, +4, hysteresis, UIP) and with final clinical results.

References

1. Suter P, Fairley HB, Isenberg MD (1978) Effect of tidal volume and positive end-expiratory pressure on compliance during mechanical ventilation. Chest 73:158–162
2. Matamis D, Lemaire F, Harf A, et al (1984) Total respiratory pressure-volume curves in the adult respiratory distress syndrome. Chest 86:58–66
3. Mankikian B, Lemaire F, Benito S, et al (1983) A new device for measurement of pulmonary pressure-volume curves in patients on mechanical ventilation. Crit Care Med 11:897–901

4. Servillo G, Svantesson C, Beydon L, et al (1997) Pressure-volume curves in acute respiratory failure. Automated low flow inflation versus occlusion. Am J Respir Crit Care Med 155:1629–1636
5. Lee WL, Stewart TE, MacDonald R, et al (2002) Safety of pressure volume curve measurement in acute lung injury and ARDS using a syringe technique. Chest 121:1595–1601
6. Gattinoni L, Pesenti A, Avalli L, et al (1987) Pressure-volume curve of total respiratory system in acute respiratory failure. Computed tomography scan study. Am J Respir Crit Care Med 136:730–736
7. Benito S, Lemaire F (1990) Pulmonary pressure-volume in acute respiratory distress syndrome in adults: role of positive end expiratory pressure. J Crit Care 5:27–34
8. Gattinoni L, Pelosi P, Suter P, et al (1998) Acute respiratory distress syndrome caused by pulmonary and extrapulmonary disease: different syndromes? Am J Respir Crit Care Med 158:3–11
9. Blanch L, Fernandez R, Benito S et al (1987) Effect of PEEP on the arterial minus end-tidal carbon dioxide gradient. Chest 92:451–454
10. Brunet F, Jeanbourquin D, Monchi M, et al (1995) Should mechanical ventilation be optimized to blood gases, lung mechanics, or thoracic CT scan? Am J Respir Crit Care Med 152:524–530
11. Jonson B, Richard JC, Straus C, Mancebo J, Lemaire F, Brochard L (1999) Pressure-volume curves and compliance in acute lung injury. Evidence of recruitment above the lower inflection point. Am J Respir Crit Care Med 159:1172–1178
12. Richard JC, Maggiore SM, Jonson B, Mancebo J, Lemaire F, Brochard L (2001) Influence of tidal volume on alveolar recruitment. Respective role of PEEP and a recruitment maneuver. Am J Respir Crit Care Med 163:1609–1613
13. Maggiore SM, Jonson B, Richard JC, Jaber S, Lemaire F, Brochard L (2001) Alveolar derecruitment at decremental positive end-expiratory pressure levels in acute lung injury. Comparison with the lower inflection point, oxygenation and compliance. Am J Respir Crit Care Med 164 795–801
14. Mancini M, Zavala E, Mancebo J, et al (2001) Mechanisms of pulmonary gas exchange improvement during a protective ventilatory strategy in acute respiratory distress syndrome. Am J Respir Crit Care Med 164:1448–1453
15. Amato MBP, Barbas CSV, Medeiros DM, et al (1998) Effect of a protective-ventilation strategy on mortality in the acute respiratory distress syndrome. N Engl J Med 338:347–354
16. Takeuchi M, Goddon S, Dolhnikoff M, et al (2002) Set positive end-expiratory pressure during protective ventilation affects lung injury. Anesthesiology 97:682–692

What are the Best Methods for Weaning Patients from Mechanical Ventilation?

S. K. Epstein

Introduction

Although invasive mechanical ventilation has beneficial effects on acute respiratory failure pathophysiology, in most instances it principally provides support while the respiratory system recovers. Invasive mechanical ventilation is associated with significant time-dependent risks and complications including ventilator-associated pneumonia (VAP), sinusitis, airway injury, thromboembolism, and gastrointestinal bleeding. Therefore, once significant clinical improvement occurs, efforts shift to rapidly removing the patient from the ventilator; a process variably referred to as weaning, liberation, or discontinuation. Fortunately, 75% of patients satisfying weaning readiness criteria tolerate their initial spontaneous breathing trial (SBT), conducted with no or minimal ventilator assistance, indicating that mechanical support is no longer required. A minority are initially intolerant of spontaneous breathing and require a more gradual weaning process. Once spontaneous breathing or weaning is tolerated, the question of whether the endotracheal tube is still required is addressed to determine suitability for extubation. A large recent body of evidence provides the basis for offering concise recommendations on the best methods for weaning from mechanical ventilation (Table 1).

Assessment of Readiness: Using Clinical Factors and "Weaning Predictors"

Rapid liberation from mechanical ventilation must be balanced against the risks of premature trials of spontaneous breathing (e.g., structural respiratory muscle injury or fatigue, cardiac dysfunction).

Assessment of readiness commences within hours for intubation related to rapidly reversible processes (e.g., cardiogenic pulmonary edema, drug overdose) while for other processes, 24–48 hours of full ventilatory support may be required before evaluating the patient for weaning. Subjective readiness criteria alone appear insufficient and have been supplemented [1, 2], or replaced [3, 4], by objective clinical assessments (e.g., evidence of clinical improvement, $PaO_2/FiO_2 \geq 150$ on positive end-expiratory pressure [PEEP] ≤ 5, adequate hemodynamics) that serve as surrogate markers of recovery. These objective assessments should serve as

Table 1. Evidence-based recommendations.

Summary Statement	Level of Evidence
Assessment of readiness for trials of spontaneous breathing should be based primarily on evidence for some clinical improvement, adequate oxygenation and hemodynamic stability.	B
The majority (~75%) of patients satisfying readiness criteria will tolerate their first spontaneous trial and do not require a slow progressive withdrawal from ventilatory support.	A
Under most circumstances weaning predictors are minimally helpful in deciding whether or not to initiate SBTs or reduce the level of ventilatory support. If a weaning predictor is to be used, the frequency-tidal volume ratio appears to be the most accurate.	B
Readiness testing is best performed with a 120-minute SBT conducted on T-piece or on low levels of CPAP or pressure support. (For the initial SBT, a 30-minute T-piece or PSV trial is adequate.)	A
Tolerance for the spontaneous breathing trial is assessed by monitoring vital signs, oximetry, gas exchange and absence of clinical signs indicative of increased work of breathing.	B
Weaning intolerance most often results from an imbalance between respiratory muscle capacity and respiratory load, cardiac dysfunction, or psychological causes. Patients failing SBTs or weaning should undergo extensive evaluation to identify reversible causes.	C
Progressive withdrawal of ventilatory support can be carried out using T-piece, pressure support or a combination of pressure support and SIMV.	B
SIMV alone should not be used for weaning.	A
Non-invasive ventilation can be used to facilitate weaning in select patients with acute on chronic respiratory failure.	B
Once a patient has passed the SBT or weaning trial, extubation should be carried out if there is adequate cough, minimal secretions, and no evidence of upper airway obstruction.	C
Upper airway obstruction should be sought in high risk patients using either the qualitative or quantitative cuff leak test.	C
Secretions should be assessed by determining the frequency of airway suctioning.	C
NIV can be used in COPD patients with early signs of extubation failure. NIV should not be used routinely after extubation or with overt post-extubation respiratory failure when intubation is immediately needed.	B
A protocol, implemented by respiratory care practitioners and ICU nurses should be used to assess daily readiness (and monitor) for spontaneous breathing trials and to direct the weaning process.	A
Protocols to decrease the use of continuous intravenous sedation reduce the duration of weaning.	A

SBT: spontaneous breathing trial; SIMV: synchronized intermittent mandatory ventilation; NIV: non-invasive ventilation; COPD: chronic obstructiove pulmonary disease; PSV: pressure support ventilation guidelines rather than rigid criteria. For example, in one large randomized controlled clinical trial, 30% of patients *never* satisfying objective readiness criteria were still ultimately weaned from mechanical ventilation [3]. Similarly, one prospective observational study and a post-hoc analysis of one randomized controlled trial show that failure to satisfy some individual readiness criteria (e.g., Glasgow Coma Scale >8, hemoglobin ≥10 mg/dl) does not preclude successful weaning [5, 6].

Recognition of important design flaws in observational studies has led to an extensive reevaluation of objective physiologic criteria ('weaning predictors') and their role in assessing weaning readiness. A comprehensive evidence-based medicine review concluded that relatively few of the more than 50 available predictors led to clinically significant changes in the probability of weaning success or failure [7, 8]. Only five predictors measured during ventilatory support (negative inspiratory force [NIF], maximum inspiratory pressure [MIP], minute ventilation, P0.1/MIP, CROP [compliance, rate, oxygenation, pressure]) have possible value in predicting weaning outcome [7, 8]. Only the latter two have likelihood ratios suggesting clinical utility, but the small number of patients studied precludes recommending their application. Accuracy is better for three additional parameters (respiratory frequency, tidal volume, frequency/tidal volume ratio [f/V_T]), measured during 1–3 minutes of unassisted breathing, but even these tests are associated with only small to moderate changes in the probability of success or failure [7, 8]. To date, there are no published randomized controlled trials specifically examining the role of weaning predictors in weaning decision making. Given the limited predicted value of weaning predictors and the inherent safety of a closely monitored SBT, a task force recommended that these tests not be routinely used [8].

Readiness Testing

After objective criteria are satisfied, formal readiness testing is conducted by a SBT on low levels of pressure support ventilation (PSV ≤ 7 mmHg), continuous positive airway pressure (CPAP), or unassisted through a T-piece. A SBT is generally mandatory because nearly 40% of patients directly extubated after satisfying readiness criteria require reintubation.

Randomized trials comparing PSV to T-piece, CPAP to T-piece, and automatic tube compensation (ATC) to PSV or T-piece have shown no differences in terms of successful weaning and extubation [9]. In one randomized controlled trial of 484 patients, the SBT failure rate tended to be higher for T-piece compared to PSV (22 v 14%), suggesting that endotracheal tube-related imposed work of breathing causes weaning failure in some patients [10]. Tolerance for 120 minutes of spontaneous breathing signals that a patient no longer requires ventilatory support [2, 3, 10–12]. Yet, two randomized controlled trials found similar rates of weaning success when comparing patients randomized to either 30- or 120 minutes of T-piece [11], or PSV breathing [13]. These investigations examined only the *first* attempt at spontaneous breathing; therefore, the ideal duration for subsequent SBTs remains unknown.

Careful assessment during the SBT is based on both objective and subjective criteria. Although these criteria are collectively widely applied [2, 3, 10–12], the individual components have not been subjected to rigorous validation to identify optimal thresholds. Post-hoc analyses of randomized controlled trials demonstrate that sequential analysis of respiratory rate, heart rate, oxygenation, and blood pressure can separate weaning failure from success patients but do not identify patients who pass the SBT but fail extubation [10, 11].

Identifying and Treating the Causes of Weaning Failure

Observational, physiologic studies demonstrate that weaning failure can result from an imbalance between respiratory load (increased work of breathing, resistive, elastic, ventilatory) and respiratory muscle capacity; imposed work of breathing, myocardial dysfunction (cardiac ischemia or congestive heart failure), or psychological factors (anxiety, delirium) [14, 15]. Therefore, intolerance for weaning trials should prompt a thorough investigation for the underlying cause with the goal of identifying, and ultimately treating, reversible factors. That said, neither observational nor randomized controlled trials have been conducted to determine if systematic identification and correction of these processes improves outcome.

Modes of Progressive Withdrawal

Once the limiting factors are addressed, further efforts to wean the patient are indicated. An area of uncertainty is the duration of rest required prior to initiating further weaning attempts. Physiologic studies indicate that respiratory muscle fatigue is infrequently detected during a failed, but well-monitored, SBT, but when present may take ≥ 24 hours to fully recover [16]. Nevertheless, one large randomized controlled trial found no difference in outcome for patients given multiple daily SBTs and those given a single daily trial (e.g., 24 hours of rest between attempts).[1]

After failing an initial SBT, patients often undergo more gradual reductions in ventilatory support (progressive withdrawal), theoretically slowly shifting work from ventilator to patient until tolerance for a minimal level of support signals that ventilatory support is no longer required. Two large multicenter randomized controlled trials directly compared different weaning techniques in patients who satisfied readiness criteria but failed to tolerate a two-hour trial of spontaneous breathing [1, 2]. Taken together, these studies indicate that a slow reduction in PSV and daily SBTs using a T-piece are equivalently efficient in weaning patients from mechanical ventilation [9]. Brochard and coworkers found that PSV reduced weaning duration compared to T-piece and synchronized intermittent mandatory ventilation (SIMV) groups (5.7 v. 9.3 days) and was more likely to be associated with weaning success [2]. Esteban et al. also incorporated a strategy of daily SBT (T-piece) with maintenance on full ventilatory support during intervening periods [1]. The T-piece (either once daily or multiple daily trials) technique shortened the median duration of mechanical ventilation when compared to progressive withdrawal with either PSV or SIMV (3 v. 4 v. 5 days) [1]. An additional major contribution of these studies was the demonstration that SIMV alone slows the process of weaning. This finding is anticipated because during lower levels of SIMV, respiratory muscle contraction is similar for both unsupported and supported breaths, indicating poor neuromuscular apparatus adaptation to changing loads [17]. Adding PSV to SIMV reduces work for both unsupported *and* supported breaths. A single, small randomized controlled trial of 19 chronic obstructive pumonary disease (COPD) patients found a trend toward shorter weaning duration among patients on SIMV/PSV compared to SIMV alone [18]. To date, no studies are available examining the utility of combining progressive withdrawal with daily SBTs.

Two randomized controlled trials indicate that non-invasive ventilation (NIV) can be used to facilitate weaning in selected patients with acute on chronic respiratory failure. Nava and colleagues randomized 50 intubated COPD patients who failed a T-piece trial to standard PSV weaning or to immediate extubation to non-invasive PSV using a full face mask and standard intensive care unit (ICU) ventilator [19]. The NIV strategy resulted in statistically significant reductions in the duration of mechanical ventilation, length of ICU stay, and 60–day survival. An additional investigation of 53 patients (approximately one half with COPD) found that NIV led to reduced duration of invasive mechanical ventilation, though other outcomes were equivalent [20]. Larger studies, including patients with other forms of respiratory failure and well-defined selection criteria are required before this technique can be generally recommended.

Extubation

Once the patient tolerates a trial of spontaneous breathing the focus shifts to determining if the endotracheal tube is still required. Approximately 2–25% of patients require reintubation (extubation failure) within 24–72h of planned extubation [21]. Most investigations demonstrate that reintubated patients suffer increased hospital mortality, prolonged ICU and hospital stays, and more frequently need long-term acute care [10, 11, 21, 22]. On the other hand, unnecessary delays in extubation prolong ICU stay, heighten the risk for pneumonia, and increase hospital mortality [5].

Standard weaning predictors are not satisfactorily accurate in predicting extubation outcome [7]. Tests designed to identify specific causes of extubation failure (excessive respiratory secretions, upper airway obstruction, inadequate cough) have been examined in prospective observational studies. For example, three of four studies found that cuff leak volumes (the difference between inspired and expired tidal volume during endotracheal tube cuff deflation) of <110 ml or <10–15% of delivered tidal volume identify patients at elevated risk for post-extubation stridor [21]. Cough effectiveness and capacity to adequately protect the airway and expel secretions have been assessed in two prospective, observational studies of brain-injured and medical-cardiac ICU patients respectively. Both investigations found that weak spontaneous cough and frequent need for airway suctioning (more often than every two hours) were predictive of extubation failure [5, 23]. The importance of adequate neurologic function for extubation success remains uncertain as two prospective observational studies in brain-injured patients arrived at opposite conclusions [5, 24].

When medical strategies fail to reverse post-extubation respiratory failure it is imperative to rapidly re-establish ventilatory support. Several prospective and retrospective observational studies noted that rapid reinstitution of invasive ventilatory support (within 12 hours of extubation) is associated with lower mortality [21]. A number of observational studies suggested that NIV was effective in preventing reintubation in two thirds of patients with extubation failure. In contrast, randomized controlled trials showed that *routine* use of NIV after extubation [25] or application in heterogeneous populations with *overt* extubation failure [26] did not decrease the need for reintubation or improve survival. A single case-control investigation observed that NIV effectively reduced the need for reintubation in COPD patients with early signs and symptoms of post-extubation hypercapnic respiratory failure [27].

Application of Weaning Protocols to Facilitate Liberation from Mechanical Ventilation

Uncontrolled studies and randomized controlled trials demonstrate improved outcome with an organized approach to weaning from mechanical ventilation (e.g., using a protocol) implemented by physicians or by respiratory care practitioners and ICU nurses. Ely and colleagues randomized 300 mechanically ventilated medical patients to either standard care or an intervention strategy that coupled a daily readiness screen with SBTs [3]. Control patients were screened without further intercession while, intervention patients passing the readiness screen underwent a two-hour SBT on CPAP or T-piece coupled with a prompt to managing clinicians encouraging extubation for those passing the SBT. The intervention strategy resulted in significant reductions in weaning time (1 vs. 3 days), duration of mechanical ventilation (4.5 v. 6 days), overall complication rate, and ICU costs. Three subsequent randomized controlled trials conducted in medical, surgical, and pediatric ICUs found that a respiratory care practitioner-ICU nurse implemented protocol shortened the duration of mechanical ventilation compared to traditional physician-directed weaning [4, 28, 29]. Despite these successes, significant questions remain on how to best implement and sustain weaning protocols, especially in unique patient populations. As an example, a daily screen/SBT strategy failed to improve outcome in a cohort of neurosurgical patients [24].

Randomized trials have demonstrated that protocols directed at minimizing the use of sedative infusions can shorten the duration of mechanical ventilation [30, 31]. Observational and case control studies indicate that a reduced duration of mechanical ventilation occurs when nurse/patient ratios improve and when a bedside weaning board and flow sheet is used to enhance communication between critical care practitioners.

References

1. Esteban A, Frutos F, Tobin MJ, et al (1995) A comparison of four methods of weaning patients from mechanical ventilation. N Engl J Med 332:345–350
2. Brochard L, Rauss A, Benito S, et al (1994) Comparison of three methods of gradual withdrawal from ventilatory support during weaning from mechanical ventilation. Am J Respir Crit Care Med 150:896–903
3. Ely EW, Baker AM, Dunagan DP, et al (1996) Effect on the duration of mechanical ventilation of identifying patients capable of breathing spontaneously. N Engl J Med 335:1864–1869
4. Kollef MH, Shapiro SD, Silver P, et al (1997) A randomized, controlled trial of protocol-directed versus physician- directed weaning from mechanical ventilation. Crit Care Med 25:567–574
5. Coplin WM, Pierson DJ, Cooley KD, et al (2000) Implications of Extubation Delay in Brain-Injured Patients Meeting Standard Weaning Criteria. Am J Respir Crit Care Med 161:1530–1536
6. Hebert PC, Blajchman MA, Cook DJ, et al (2001) Do blood transfusions improve outcomes related to mechanical ventilation? Chest 119:1850–1857
7. Meade M, Guyatt G, Cook D, et al (2001) Predicting success in weaning from mechanical ventilation. Chest 120:400S–424S
8. MacIntyre N, Cook D, Ely E, et al (2001) Evidence-based guidelines for weaning and discontinuing ventilatory support: A collective Task Force facilitated by the American College of Chest Physicians; the American Association for Respiratory Care; and the American College of Critical Care Medicine. Chest 120:375S–396S
9. Meade M, Guyatt G, Sinuff T, et al (2001) Trials Comparing Alternative Weaning Modes and Discontinuation Assessments. Chest 120:425S–437S
10. Esteban A, Alia I, Gordo F, et al (1997) Extubation outcome after spontaneous breathing trials with t-tube or pressure support ventilation. Am J Respir Crit Care Med. 156:459–465
11. Esteban A, Alia I, Tobin M, et al (1999) Effect of spontaneous breathing trial duration on outcome of attempts to discontinue mechanical ventilation. Am J Respir Crit Care Med 159:512–518
12. Vallverdu I, Calaf N, Subirana M, et al (1998) Clinical characteristics, respiratory functional parameters, and outcome of two-hour t-piece trial in patients weaning from mechanical ventilation. Am J Respir Crit Care Med 158:1855–1862
13. Perren A, Domenighetti G, Mauri S, et al (2002) Protocol-directed weaning from mechanical ventilation: clinical outcome in patients randomized for a 30-min or 120-min trial with pressure support ventilation. Intensive Care Med 28:1058–1063
14. Jubran A, Tobin MJ (1997) Pathophysiologic basis of acute respiratory distress in patients who fail a trial of weaning from mechanical ventilation. Am J Respir Crit Care Med 155:906–915
15. Lemaire F, Teboul JL, Cinotti L, et al (1988) Acute left ventricular dysfunction during unsuccessful weaning from mechanical ventilation. Anesthesiology 69:171–179
16. Laghi F, D'Alfonso N, Tobin MJ (1995) Pattern of recovery from diaphragmatic fatigue over 24 hours. J Appl Physiol 79:539–546
17. Imsand C, Feihl F, Perret C, et al (1994) Regulation of inspiratory neuromuscular output during synchronized intermittent mechanical ventilation. Anesthesiology 80:13–22
18. Jounieaux V, Duran A, Levi-Valensi P (1994) Synchronized intermittent mandatory ventilation with and without pressure support ventilation in weaning patients with COPD from mechanical ventilation. Chest 105:1204–1210
19. Nava S, Ambrosino N, Clini E (1998) Noninvasive mechanical ventilation in the weaning of patients with respiratory failure due to chronic obstructive pulmonary disease. A randomized, controlled trial. Ann Intern Med 128:721–728

20. Girault C, Daudenthun I, Chevron V, et al (1999) Noninvasive ventilation as a systematic extubation and weaning technique in acute-on-chronic respiratory failure. A prospective, randomized controlled study. Am J Respir Crit Care Med 160:86–92
21. Epstein SK (2002) Decision to extubate. Intensive Care Med 28:535–546
22. Epstein SK, Ciubotaru RL, Wong JB (1997) Effect of failed extubation on the outcome of mechanical ventilation. Chest 112:186–192
23. Khamiees M, Raju P, DeGirolamo A, et al (2001) Predictors of extubation outcome in patients who have successfully completed a spontaneous breathing trial. Chest 120:1262–1270
24. Namen AM, Ely EW, Tatter SB, et al (2001) Predictors of successful extubation in neurosurgical patients. Am J Respir Crit Care Med 163:658–664
25. Jiang J, Kao S, Wang S (1999) Effect of early application of biphasic positive airway pressure on the outcome of extubation in ventilatory weaning. Respirology 4:161–165
26. Keenan SP, Powers C, McCormack DG, et al (2002) Noninvasive positive-pressure ventilation for postextubation respiratory distress: a randomized controlled trial. JAMA 287:3238–3244
27. Hilbert G, Gruson D, Portel L, et al (1998) Noninvasive pressure support ventilation in COPD patients with postextubation hypercapnic respiratory insufficiency. Eur Respir J. 11:1349–1353
28. Marelich GP, Murin S, Battistella F, Inciardi J, Viera T, Roby M (2000) Protocol weaning of mechanical ventilation in medical and surgical patients by respiratory care practitioners and nurses: effect on weaning time and incidence of ventilator-associated pneumonia. Chest 118:459–467
29. Schultz TR, Lin RJ, Watzman HM, et al (2001) Weaning children from mechanical ventilation: a prospective randomized trial of protocol-directed versus physician-directed weaning. Respir Care 46:772–782
30. Brook AD, Ahrens TS, Schaiff R, et al (1999) Effect of a nursing-implemented sedation protocol on the duration of mechanical ventilation. Crit Care Med 27:2609–2615
31. Kress JP, Pohlman AS, O'Connor MF, et al (2000) Daily interruption of sedative infusions in critically ill patients undergoing mechanical ventilation. N Engl J Med 342:1471–1477

Venous Thromboembolism in the ICU: What is the Epidemiology and What are the Consequences?

D. Cook, M. Crowther, and M. Meade

Introduction

Venous thromboembolism (VTE) is a common complication of critical illness, conferring considerable morbidity and mortality in hospitalized patients. Patients with deep venous thrombosis (DVT) are at risk of developing pulmonary embolism (PE) which may be fatal. Approximately 90% of cases of DVT leading to PE are believed to arise in the lower extremities.

In one study, PE was found at autopsy in 59 of 404 hospitalized patients (14.6%, 95% CI 11.3–18.4%), and PE was unsuspected in 14/20 patients who died from PE (70.0%, 95% CI 45.7–88.1%) [1]. In one longitudinal study over 25 years, 9% of autopsies identified PE, and in 84% of patients, the clinical diagnosis was missed [2]. In a clinical study highlighting this problem in practice, 13/34 (38.2%) of ICU patients with known DVT who had no symptoms of PE were diagnosed with PE by ventilation-perfusion scans [3]. We posit that in critically ill patients with impaired cardiopulmonary reserve, a small PE, which might be of minimal clinical importance in less ill patients, might have severe or fatal consequences. It is possible that many mechanically ventilated patients with sudden episodes of hypotension, tachycardia, or hypoxia may have undetected PE. The contribution of PE to difficulty weaning patients from mechanical ventilation has been also questioned [4].

The clinical importance of DVT in medical-surgical ICU patients lies primarily in its association with PE, and in the fact that DVT is more easily diagnosed than PE. Thus, the consequences of DVT have the potential to be particularly serious, yet paradoxically, unrecognized in ICU patients. Concern about undiagnosed VTE in the ICU is heightened by research showing that 10 [5] to100% [4, 6] of DVTs found by ultrasound screening were clinically unsuspected (Evidence Category C).

Risk Factors for VTE

Understanding the epidemiology of VTE requires knowledge of VTE risk factors. Inherited and acquired abnormalities in coagulation predispose to VTE. The two most common abnormalities in the coagulation cascade associated with VTE are the factor V Leiden mutation and the prothrombin 20210A regulatory sequence mutation. Additional inherited procoagulant states include deficiencies of protein

C, protein S and antithrombin, each of which are naturally occurring anticoagulant proteins, and elevations in the levels of homocysteine, and coagulation factors VIII, IX and XI.

When compared to general hospital patients or outpatients, critically ill patients have an increased risk of DVT due to immobility, sedation, paralysis [7], and activation of the inflammatory and coagulation cascades. Using primarily univariate analyses and some multivariate analyses, studies in medical-surgical ICU patients have identified VTE predictors in the intensive care unit (ICU) [4, 8–10]. These include patient demographics (e.g., female sex), prior VTE, recent morbidity (e.g., duration of pre-ICU hospital stay), ICU procedures (e.g., central venous catheters), treatments (e.g., mechanical ventilation), and lack of use of prophylaxis (decreasing risk). These studies have yielded some useful risk factor information; the findings underscore how some risk factors are present at baseline and immutable (e.g., personal history) while others are modifiable (e.g., central venous catheterization).

In summary, VTE is a multicausal disease. However, no studies have been designed to analyze the influence of, and interaction among, genetic markers, premorbid illnesses and events and exposures that predispose to VTE among mechanically ventilated patients (Evidence Category C).

Diagnosis of VTE

A key issue in understanding the epidemiology of VTE is knowing the incidence of DVT. The incidence of DVT is dependent upon the diagnostic method employed, since different detection methods yield different incidence rates. In terms of the physical examination, a helpful constellation of signs and symptoms in a mathematically derived and validated clinical model has been shown to predict DVT in both outpatients and non-critically ill inpatients [11]. However, diagnosing DVT in the ICU is more challenging. Symptoms are rarely elicited from mechanically ventilated patients, most of whom receive sedation and analgesia. The physical examination tends not to receive the same priority by ICU clinicians as cardiorespiratory monitoring devices. Therefore, basing our understanding of the epidemiology of DVT on events detected by the clinical history and physical examination is unsuitable.

The reference standard for DVT remains lower extremity venography. Venography is highly sensitive for DVTs including those poorly seen by ultrasound (localized, non-occlusive or pelvic); venography is the only reliable test to detect calf vein thrombus. However, venography is rarely performed in ICU patients [12]. Concern about transporting potentially unstable patients to the Radiology Department, the invasivenes of the test, and the risk of contrast dye-induced nephropathy may also contribute to aversion to venography in this setting. Bilateral lower extremity compression Doppler ultrasound is the most widely used diagnostic test for DVT according to our Canadian survey [12], a survey of UK radiologists [13], and VTE researchers in the medical-surgical ICU population [4, 6, 14]. A meta-analysis reported a pooled sensitivity of Doppler ultrasound for proximal DVTs in symptomatic patients of 97% (95%CI 96–98%) and in asymptomatic patients, 62%

(95%CI 53–71%) [15]. The test properties of ultrasonography for DVT in mechanically ventilated ICU patients have not been determined.

Since the likelihood of embolization from undiagnosed, untreated proximal DVT is high, strategies which screen for proximal DVT in this critically ill population have the potential to reduce the risk of PE and its cardiopulmonary consequences through early treatment. However, we have no diagnostic test for DVT that has been demonstrated to be both accurate and feasible for daily practice in mechanically ventilated patients. Universal screening for DVT with ultrasonography, although the most widely accepted DVT diagnostic test in this setting, cannot be recommended due to the absence of evidence about its impact on clinically important outcomes (Evidence Category C and D). The properties of various diagnostic tests for PE are summarized elsewhere, but no studies have rigorously evaluated their properties in the ICU setting (Evidence Category D) .

Incidence of VTE

A key point about the epidemiology of VTE is that the incidence is dependent on the population of ICU patients evaluated as well as the diagnostic method employed. Thus, across-study comparisons about the incidence of VTE are problematic. Nevertheless, some critically ill populations have a high rate of VTE compared to other populations; in this sense, the subpopulation of critically ill patients is also a risk factor for VTE. For example, in a study of screening ultrasonography, among 716 trauma patients who did not receive prophylaxis, 349 adequate venograms were performed; 58% (95%CI 52–63%) of patients had DVT between days 14–21, of which one third were proximal [16]. Medical-surgical ICU patients have a mid-range risk of VTE, lower than trauma and neurosurgery patients, but higher than ward medical or surgical patients. A schematic showing risk stratification is found in Figure 1.

VTE Prophylaxis

Multiple lines of evidence support the principle that prophylaxis reduces the risk of VTE in patients at risk [17]. A systematic review of randomized trials of VTE prophylaxis included several critically ill populations [7]. Trauma patients have a lower rate of DVT when receiving low molecular weight heparin (LMWH) compared to unfractionated heparin. One randomized trial in trauma patients found that 31% of patients receiving enoxaparin developed DVT compared to 44% in the heparin group (relative risk reduction 30%) [18] (Evidence Category A). Pooling all studies comparing either unfractionated heparin or LMWH against mechanical approaches to prophylaxis, the pooled odds ratio is 0.46 (95%CI 0.16–1.29) favouring anticoagulants (Evidence Category A). For neurosurgical patients, pooling data from 5 randomized trials comparing mechanical approaches to no prophylaxis yields an odds ratio of 0.28 (95% CI 0.17–0.46) in favour of mechanical prophylaxis (Evidence Category A). Pooling the results of three trials comparing combined LWMH and mechanical approaches versus mechanical alone yields a

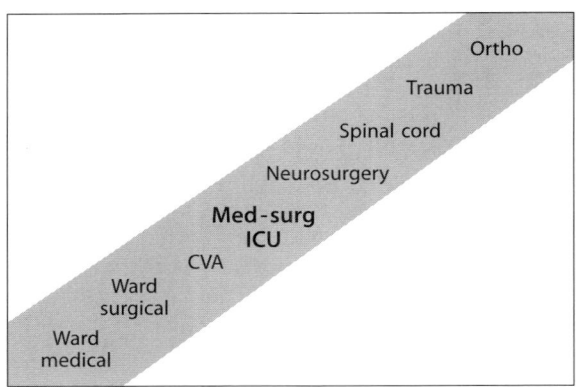

Fig. 1. Risk of VTE in the ICU

pooled odds ratio of 0.59 (95% CI 0.40–0.85) favoring combination prophylaxis (Evidence Category A).

One large randomized trial of acutely ill medical patients demonstrated that LMWH was associated with lower DVT rates than placebo; however, this trial excluded patients requiring mechanical ventilation [19]. Considering mechanically ventilated patients, two randomized trials have tested DVT prophylaxis in the medical-surgical ICU. One double blind trial allocated 119 medical-surgical ICU patients at least 40 years of age to unfractionated heparin 5,000 IU twice daily or placebo [20]. Using serial fibrinogen leg scanning for 5 days, the rates of DVT were 13% in the heparin group and 29% in the placebo group (relative risk reduction 0.65). Rates of bleeding and PE were not reported. In a second multicenter trial by Fraisse and colleagues [21], 223 patients with an acute exacerbation of COPD requiring mechanical ventilation for at least 2 days were allocated to nadroparin 3,800 or 5,700 IU once daily, or placebo. Weekly duplex ultrasound was used to screen for DVT, and venography was attempted in all patients. The DVT rate was 16% in the nadroparin group and 28% in the placebo group (relative risk reduction 0.45). A similar number of patients bled (25 vs 18 patients, respectively, p=0.18). In summary, both unfractionated heparin and LMWH provide effective VTE prophylaxis in the medical-surgical ICU population (Evidence Category A)., although no trials have compared these approaches.

Finally, the incidence of VTE is dependent on the extent to which VTE prophylaxis is applied. One cross-sectional utilization review showed that mechanically ventilated surgical patients are less likely to receive VTE prophylaxis than surgical patients who are spontaneously breathing, perhaps reflecting concern about maintaining hemostasis following heparin administration in the immediate post operative period [22]. Early utilization reviews have indicated insufficient application of VTE prophylaxis, but recent studies suggest that attention to VTE prevention is increasing [22, Lacherade, unpublished data], which should decrease the burden of illness of VTE in mechanically ventilated patients (Evidence Category C).

References

1. Stein PD, Henry JW (1995) Prevalence of acute pulmonary embolism among patients in a general hospital and at autopsy. Chest 108:978–981
2. Karwinski B, Svendsen E (1989) Comparison of clinical and postmortem diagnosis of pulmonary embolism. J Clin Pathol 42:135–139
3. Moser KM, Fedullo PF, LittleJohn JK, Crawford R (1994) Frequent asymptomatic pulmonary embolism in patients with deep venous thrombosis. JAMA 271:223–225
4. Hirsch DR, Ingenito EP, Goldhaber SZ (1995) Prevalence of deep venous thrombosis among patients in medical intensive care. JAMA 274:335–337
5. Marik PE, Andrews L, Maini B (1997) The incidence of deep venous thrombosis in ICU patients. Chest 111:661–664
6. Harris LM, Curl RC, Booth FV, Hassett JM, Leney G, Ricotta JJ (1997) Screening for asymptomatic deep vein thrombosis in surgical intensive care patients. J Vasc Surg 26:764–769
7. Attia J, Ray JG, Cook DJ, Douketis J, Ginsberg JS, Geerts W (2001) Deep vein thrombosis and its prevention in critically ill patients. Arch Intern Med 161:1268–1279
8. Kollef MH, Eisenberg PR, Shannon W (1998) A rapid assay for the detection of circulating D-dimer is associated with clinical outcomes among critically ill patients. Crit Care Med 26:1054–1060
9. Cook DJ, Attia J, Weaver B, McDonald E, Meade M, Crowther M (2000) Venous thromboembolic disease: An observational study in medical-surgical intensive care unit patients. J Crit Care 15:127–132
10. Nbrahim EH, Iregul M, Prentice D, Sherman G, Kollef MH, Shannon W (2002) Deep vein thrombosis during prolonged mechanical ventilation. Crit Care Med 30:771–774
11. Wells PS, Anderson DR, Bormanis J, et al (1999) Application of a diagnostic clinical model for the management of hospitalized patients with suspected deep-vein thrombosis. Thromb Haemost 81:493–497
12. Cook DJ, McMullin J, Hodder R, et al (2001) Prevention and diagnosis of venous thromboembolism in critically ill patients: A Canadian survey. Crit Care 5:336–342
13. Burn PR, Blunt DM, Sansom HE, Phelan MS (1997) The radiological investigation of suspected lower limb deep vein thrombosis. Clin Radiol 52:625–628
14. Moser KM, LeMoine JR, Nachtwey FJ, Spragg RG (1981) Deep venous thrombosis and pulmonary embolism. Frequency in a respiratory intensive care unit. JAMA 246:1422–1424
15. Kearon C, Julian JA, Newman TE, Ginsberg JS (1998) Noninvasive diagnosis of deep venous thrombosis. McMaster Diagnostic Imaging Practice Guidelines Initiative. Ann Intern Med 128:563–677
16. Geerts WH, Code KI, Jay RM, Chen E, Szalai JP (1994) A prospective study of venous thromboembolism after major trauma. N Engl J Med 331:1601–1606
17. Geerts WH, Heit JA, Clagett P, et al (2001) Prevention of venous thromboembolism. Sixth ACCP Antithrombotic Consensus Conference on Antithrombotic Therapy. Chest 119:132S–175S
18. Geerts WH, Jay RM, Code KI, et al (1996) A comparison of low-dose heparin with low-molecular weight heparin as prophylaxis against venous thromboembolism after major trauma. N Engl J Med 335:701–707
19. Samama MM, Cohen AT, Darmon JY, et al (1999) A comparison of enoxaparin versus placebo for the prevention of venous thromboembolism in acutely ill medical patients. Prophylaxis in Medical Patients with Enoxaparin Group. N Engl J Med 341:793–800
20. Cade JF (1982) High risk of the critically ill for venous thromboembolism. Crit Care Med 10:448–450
21. Fraisse F, Holzapfel L, Couland JM, et al (2000) Nadroparin in the prevention of deep vein thrombosis in acute decompensated COPD. Association of Non-University Affiliated Intensive Care Specialist Physicians in France. Am J Respir Crit Care Med 161:1109–1114

22. Cook DJ, Laporta D, Skrobik Y, et al (2001) Prevention of venous thromboembolism in critically ill surgery patients: A cross-sectional study. J Crit Care 16:161–166

Non-invasive Ventilation:
How, when, for whom, and what outcome?

L. Brochard

Introduction

Restricting the benefit of clinical research to randomized clinical trials would be a mistake in the field of non-invasive ventilation (NIV). Observational studies, physiological studies, and matched paired case-control studies have put together an enormous body evidence demonstrating the benefits of NIV and the working mechanisms of this technique. The randomized controlled trials have confirmed the evidence and helped to more formally indicate when NIV should be a first line treatment. Randomized controlled trials, however, are non-blinded, are highly selective regarding the inclusion of patients, and do not represent the real life. Additional studies conducted out of the context of clinical trials are of utmost importance to ensure that the results of these trials can be observed in real life.

In this chapter, the main studies focusing on the efficacy of NIV in acute respiratory failure will be reviewed. Articles published in non-English language and meta-analysis will not be considered. When data are available, the discussion will address the type of ventilatory modality.

Non-invasive Ventilation in Acute Exacerbation
of Chronic Respiratory Failure (Table 1)

The studies including acute on chronic respiratory failure most frequently concern patients with chronic obstructive pulmonary disease (COPD). Definitions for chronic diseases, however, are sometimes imprecise.

Patients with hypercapnic forms of acute respiratory failure are most likely to benefit from NIV. The pathophysiology of most episodes of acute decompensation of chronic respiratory failure was demonstrated in a physiological study [1], and involves the inability of respiratory muscles to generate adequate alveolar ventilation in the presence of severe abnormalities in respiratory mechanics (intrinsic positive end-expiratory pressure [PEEP], high inspiratory resistances). Therefore, despite massive stimulation of the respiratory centres and large negative intrathoracic pressure swings generated by the respiratory muscles, these patients generate small tidal volumes at the mouth, which are inadequately compensated for by an increase in breathing rate [1]. This rapid shallow breathing has limited efficiency for removing CO_2 and is associated with a potential risk of respiratory

Table 1. Main studies of the efficacy of non-invasive ventilation (NIV) in patients with chronic obstructive pulmonary disease (COPD)

Author, year [ref] Number of pts	Population/ Location	Type of study	Conclusions for NIV
Brochard, 1990 [1] n = 26	COPD/ICU	Case control study	Reduction of ETI, length of stay
Vitacca, 1993 [7] n = 29	COPD/ICU . RCT PSV vs ACV . Cohort (35)		The two modalities had better results than conventional treatment
Bott, 1993 [6] n = 60	COPD/ward	**RCT**	Improvement of ABG, dyspnea Reduction of ETI criteria Reduction in mortality (after excluding 4 patients who did not receive NIV)
Kramer, 1995 [8] n = 31	Mixed 74 % of COPD/ICU	RCT	Improvement of ABG, dyspnea Reduction of ETI (67 % to 9 % in COPD)
Brochard, 1995 [9] n = 84	COPD/ICU	RCT	Improvement of ABG Reduction of ETI (74 % to 26 %), of complications, LOS Reduction in mortality
Barbé, 1996 [21] n= 24	COPD/ emergency ward	RCT	No benefit of NIV **Note:** *no patient required ETI*
Angus, 1996 [10] n = 17	COPD NIV vs doxapram	RCT	Improvement in ABG
Celikel, 1998 [11] n = 30	COPD	RCT	Improvement of ABG Reduction of criteria for ETI, of LOS
Confalonieri, 1999 [40] n = 56	Community-acquired pneumonia – 41% of COPD/ICU	RCT	Improvement of ABG Reduction of ETI (50 % to 21 %), of complications, of ICU stay Improvement in 2 month survival for COPD (38% vs 89 %)
Plant, 2000 [12] n = 236	COPD / ward	RCT	Improvement of ABG Reduction of criteria for ETI Reduction in mortality
Girou, 2000 [45] n = 100	COPD and cardiogenic pulmonary edema/ICU	Case / control study	Reduction in complications (infections) and in mortality

Table 1. *Continued*

Author, year [ref] Number of pts	Population/ Location	Type of study	Conclusions for NIV
Conti, 2002 [15] n = 49	COPD admitted to the ICU (late NIV) need for ventilation:	RCT	Reduction of ETI (48 % vs 100%) Similar ICU outcome Fewer long-term readmissions (65 % vs 100 %)

Long-term follow-up

Vitacca, 1996 [16] n = 57	COPD	NonR CT	Better survival at one year follow-up (30% vs 63%)
Confalonieri, 1996 [18] n = 48	COPD	Casecontrol study	Better survival at one year follow-up (50 % vs 71 %)
Bardi, 2000 [17] n = 30	COPD	NonR CT	Better survival at one year follow-up

Post-extubation

Hilbert, 1998 [55] n = 60	COPD with post extubation respiratory distress	Case-control study	Reduction in ETI
Nava, 1998 [59] n = 50	Deliberate shortening of MV after 48 hours	RCT	Improvement of weaning success Reduction of LOS, of complications Reduction in mortality
Girault, 1999 [60] n = 33	Deliberate shortening of MV after 4–5 days	RCT	Feasibility No change in outcome Longer duration of ventilation with NIV
Carlucci, 2002 [58]	COPD with post extubation respiratory distress	RCT	Lower ETI rate (6 vs 25%) Reduction of LOS and mortality (9 vs 35%)

MV: mechanical ventilation; *ETI*: endotracheal intubation; *RCT*: randomized controlled trial; non *RCT*: non-randomized controlled trial; *LOS*: length of stay; *ICU*: Intensive care unit; *PSV*: pressure support ventilation; *ACV*: Assist-control ventilation; *ABG*: Arterial blood gases muscle fatigue. During these episodes, severe gas exchange deterioration accompanies a worsening of the clinical condition, with dyspnea, right ventricular failure, and encephalopathy. This vicious circle can be stopped by NIV, which allows the patient to take deeper breaths with less effort [1, 2]. NIV with two levels of pressure (pressure support [PSV] and PEEP) delivers a positive inspiratory pressure in synchrony with the patient's inspiratory effort, while maintaining a lower level of pressure during expiration allows to counterbalance the effects of dynamic hyperinflation, which result in a positive residual alveolar pressure at the end of expiration.

Several studies have demonstrated that NIV reverses the clinical abnormalities related to hypoxemia, hypercapnia, and acidosis [1, 3].

Clinical Trials Evaluating Need of Intubation And Outcome

Acute exacerbation of COPD is a frequent reason for hospital and ICU admission, and the efficacy of NIV in this situation has been extensively studied. A recent international consensus conference recommended that NIV be considered as a first-line treatment in these patients [4] and the British Thoracic Society Guidelines recommend that every hospital should be able to deliver NIV on a 24 hour-a-day basis in this indication [5]. In 1990, a case-control study had first demonstrated that NIV could markedly reduce the need for endotracheal intubation [1]. Subsequently, several prospective randomized trials confirmed that NIV reduces the need for endotracheal intubation and the rate of complications, shortens length of stay, and improves survival in patients with COPD [6-11]. A major reduction in the need for endotracheal intubation was found by Kramer et al. [8]. In this study, 74% of patients had COPD and the reduction in intubation rate in this group was from 67 to 9%. Two studies, conducted in the United Kingdom, showed the efficacy of NIV out of the ICU [6, 12]. In the largest study in the ICU, in which 85 patients with COPD were randomized to treatment with or without facemask PSV [9], the endotracheal intubation rate was 74% in the controls with standard medical treatment as compared to only 26% in the NIV group. This reduction was associated with fewer complications during the ICU stay, a reduced length of hospital stay, and, more importantly, a significant reduction in mortality rate (from 29 to 9%). The overall decrease in mortality was ascribable to reductions in the need for endotracheal intubation and in various ICU-related complications. A prospective, multicenter randomized trial conducted in the UK by Plant et al. compared standard therapy alone (control group) with NIV in 236 COPD patients admitted to general respiratory wards for acute respiratory failure [12]. The failure rate (reaching criteria for ETI) was higher in the control group (27% vs. 15%), and NIV was associated with a lower in-hospital mortality rate. Because of admission policy in the UK, all patients who failed NIV were not transferred to an ICU and for this reason the results may not be extrapolated to all kinds of medical institution. The authors stressed the fact that for the most severe patients (pH <7.30 on admission) the benefit of delivering NIV out of the ICU became marginal, with a high mortality rate. These patients would probably have benefited from an early ICU admission for timing NIV delivery.

These studies indicate that early NIV to prevent further deterioration must become an important part of the first-line therapy of acute exacerbation of COPD [13].

A very low pH, marked alteration in mental status when NIV is started, and presence of comorbidities or a high severity score characterize patients who experience NIV failure [14]. Several of these factors seem to indicate that a late delivery of NIV in the course of the exacerbation reduces the likelihood of success. Every effort should be made to deliver NIV early and close monitoring is, therefore, in order when NIV is started late. In addition, a recently published randomized controlled trial indicates that the efficacy of NIV is diminished when this therapy is applied lately in the course of the exacerbation. Indeed, Conti et al. showed a reduction of intubation from 100 to 52%, which was associated with only marginal short-term benefits. NIV was applied to patients with COPD who had stayed a mean of 14 hours in the emergency ward before being admitted to the ICU at the time they needed intubation [15]. Interestingly, there were still significant long-term benefits associated with the use of NIV such as a decrease in the readmission rate.

Clinical trials Evaluating Long-term Survival

Three studies have suggested that the use of NIV is associated with a better one-year survival compared to a standard ICU therapy [16, 17] or compared to invasive mechanical ventilation [18].

Clinical Trials Evaluating Location of Application of NIV

The two studies by Bott et al. and by Plant et al. were performed in the respiratory ward, with a training period of 8 hours over the three months preceding the study for the latter study [6, 12]. During the study, one hour per month on average was deemed necessary in each center to maintain the level of expertise of the personnel. One study was performed in the emergency ward but patients included had a very low severity [21]. In another study in the emergency ward, some patients with COPD were included [22]. The results of this study suggested that NIV could have inappropriately delayed endotracheal intubation. However, the small samples in this study, some imbalance between groups, and the lack of precise description of NIV settings make it difficult to draw conclusion from this study.

The feasibility of treating patients with COPD out of the ICU has been demonstrated, but applicability of the results need to take into account the need for training personnel.

Other management strategies associated with NIV

1. Negative pressure ventilation: This technique is only available in very few centers in the world. Its efficacy for treatment of acute exacerbations of COPD

seems to be superior in terms of outcome than a traditional approach with invasive mechanical ventilation [19], and may be similar to face mask NIV [20].
2. Helium-oxygen mixture: The use of a helium-oxygen mixture seems very promising during NIV in patients with COPD [23, 24]. Several randomized controlled trials are in progress to test the hypothesis that this gas mixture could increase the success rate of this technique.

Non-invasive Ventilation in Cardiogenic Pulmonary Edema (Table 2)

Studies mixed patients with different etiologies for cardiac failure. The results may differ, however, in case of ischemic heart failure

Continuous positive airway pressure (CPAP) raises intrathoracic pressure, decreases shunting, and improves arterial oxygenation and dyspnea in these patients [25]. Interestingly, CPAP can lessen the work of breathing substantially and improve cardiovascular function by decreasing the left ventricular afterload in non-preload-dependent patients [26]. Pressure support plus PEEP induces similar pathophysiological benefits.

Most patients with cardiogenic pulmonary edema improve rapidly under medical therapy. A few, however, develop acute asphyxic respiratory distress and require ventilatory support until the medical treatment starts to work. This may be particularly common in elderly patients with heart disease and in patients with concomitant chronic lung disease [27]. Several NIV modalities have been tried successfully, the goal being to avoid endotracheal intubation.

Clinical Trials Comparing CPAP or Pressure Support Plus PEEP

Randomized trials comparing either CPAP or pressure support plus PEEP to standard medical therapy found closely similar results with the two techniques in terms of improvement in arterial blood gases and breathing rate. Both CPAP and pressure support plus PEEP significantly reduced the endotracheal intubation rate rate [25, 28-30]. Two studies, however, indicate a need for caution. One compared pressure support plus PEEP and CPAP [31]. Acute myocardial infarction was more common in the pressure support plus PEEP group than in the CPAP group and it remains unclear whether this should be ascribed to a randomization bias or to a deleterious effect of pressure support plus PEEP itself. A higher rate of acute myocardial infarction was not found in the NIV arm of a randomized controlled trial with pressure support and PEEP, nor in the observational studies [32, 33]. The second study compared intravenous bolus therapy of high-dose nitrates, to conventional medical therapy (a different medical therapy) and pressure support plus PEEP. The first of these two treatments was far more effective clinically than NIV and resulted in a better outcome [34]. These two studies draw attention to the vulnerability of patients with cardiogenic pulmonary edema, particularly those with ischemic heart disease. They indicate that both appropriate drug therapy and

Table 2. Main studies of the efficacy of non-invasive ventilation (NIV) in patients with cardiogenic pulmonary edema

Author, year [ref] Number of patients	Mode of ventilation	Type of study	Conclusions for NIV
Rasanen, 1985 [28] n = 40	CPAP	RCT	Improvement in physiological parameters in "treatment failure" Reduction of ETI (65% vs 35%, p = 0.06)
Bersten, 1991 [29] n = 39	CPAP	RCT	Improvement in physiological parameters Reduction of ETI (35 % to 0%) and ICU stay
Lin, 1995 [25] n = 100	CPAP	Case control study	Improvement in physiological parameters Reduction in "treatment failure criteria" and ETI
Mehta, 1997 [31] n = 27	CPAP vs PSV + PEEP	RCT	Larger improvement in physiological parameters with PSV Higher rate of AMI with PSV (71% vs 38%)
Rustherholtz, 1999 [32] n = 26	PSV + PEEP	Cohort	Low failure rate (21 %). Success in hypercapnic patients. Failure for AMI patients
Hoffmann, 1999 [33] n = 29	PSV + PEEP	Cohort	Low failure rate (1/29)
Masip, 2000 [30] n = 40	PSV + PEEP	RCT	Improvement in physiological parameters Reduction of ETI (5% vs 33 %) and ICU stay
Sharon, 2000 [34] n = 40	PSV + PEEP Vs High doses of nitrates	RCT	More ETI and complications with NIV (85% vs 25% of failure) Note: medical therapy was different

MV: mechanical ventilation; *ETI*: endotracheal intubation; *RCT*: randomized controlled trial; non RCT: non-randomized controlled trial; *LOS*: length of stay; *ICU*: Intensive care unit; *PSV*: pressure support ventilation; *ACV*: Assist-control ventilation; *ABG*: Arterial blood gases; *PEEP*: positive end-expiratory pressure; *CPAP*: continuous positive airway pressure; *AMI*: acute myocardial infarction.

close monitoring are in order when using any form of NIV, especially in patients with ischemic heart disease.

Ventilatory support seems to be a useful adjunct to medical treatment in case of asphyxic pulmonary edema, but caution is needed in case of ischemic heart failure when using NIV.

Non-invasive Ventilation in Hypoxemic Respiratory Failure (Table 3)

The studies include very different etiologies causing hypoxemic respiratory failure.

Clinical Trials Evaluating CPAP

A recent investigation evaluated whether facemask CPAP produced physiologic benefits and reduced the need for endotracheal intubation in patients with acute lung injury (ALI) [35]. Despite an early favorable physiological response to CPAP in terms of comfort and oxygenation, no differences were found in the need for endotracheal intubation, in-hospital mortality, or length of ICU stay. In addition, the use of CPAP was associated with more complications, including stress ulcer bleeding and cardiac arrest at the time of endotracheal intubation. These results suggest that CPAP alone cannot be recommended to avoid endotracheal intubation in patients with ALI. Its use should be limited to a short initial period of time if no other method is available.

Clinical Trials Evaluating Pressure Support and PEEP

Until the late 1990s, the most convincing successes with NIV were obtained in patients with acute respiratory acidosis in whom hypoxemia was not the main reason for respiratory failure. One randomized controlled trial by Wysocki et al. found no benefit of NIV in patients with no previous history of chronic lung disease, except in the subgroup of patients who developed acute hypercapnia [36]. However, the beneficial results of NIV have now been extended to different forms of hypoxemic respiratory failure with carefully selected patients [37-39]. Recently, studies have shown that, in selected patients, NIV may reduce the need for intubation and improve outcomes [37-42]. One randomized controlled study by Antonelli et al., showed marked benefits of NIV using pressure support and PEEP in hypoxemic patients free from COPD, hemodynamic instability or neurological impairment, who were randomized when they reached pre-defined criteria for intubation [37]. Improvements in oxygenation were similar with the non-invasive or the invasive approach. Despite a 30% failure rate, patients treated with NIV had shorter duration of ventilation and ICU stay and experienced fewer complications. Thus, NIV can be effective in selected patients with hypoxemic respiratory failure but with no hemodynamic or mental impairment. Other randomized con-

Table 3. Main studies of the efficacy of non-invasive ventilation (NIV) in patients with hypoxemic respiratory failure

Author, year [ref] Number of pts	Population/ Location/Mode of ventilation	Type of study	Conclusions for NIV
Wysocki, 1995 [36] n = 41	COPD/ICU	Case-control study	No benefit of NIV Except in the sub-group with acute hypercapnia (n = 17)
Wood, 1998 [22] n = 27	RCT/ Emergency department	RCT	No benefit of NIV Trends for poorer outcome (p=0.1) Note: imbalance in randomisation, small samples
Antonelli, 1998 [37] n = 64	ALI/ICU/PSV + PEEP	RCT	Improvement of ABG Reduction of ETI (10/32 vs 100%), of complications, ICU stay Trends for better survival
Antonelli, 2000 [38] n = 40	Organ transplant/ ICU/ PSV + PEEP	RCT	Improvement of ABG Reduction of ETI (20% vs 70%), of complications Reduction in ICU mortality (20% vs 50%)
Delclaux, 2001 [35] n = 123	ALI/ICU/CPAP	RCT	No benefit of CPAP More adverse events (p = 0.01)
Martin, 2001 [39] n = 61	Mixed/ICU/ PSV + PEEP	RCT	Improvement of ABG Reduction of ETI (21 % to 6% ETI/100 days), of LOS
Hilbert, 2001] [41] n = 52	Cancer, hematologic malignancies/ ICU/PSV + PEEP	RCT	Improvement of ABG Reduction of ETI (77% to 41%), of complications Reduction in ICU and hospital mortality (81% to 50%)
Azoulay, 2001 [46] n = 237	Cancer, hematologic malignancies/ ICU/PSV + PEEP	Cohort, case-control study	Reduction of ETI, improved survival
Auriant, 2001 [49] n = 48	Lung surgery/ ICU/PSV + PEEP	RCT	Improvement of ABG Reduction of ETI (50% to 21 %), of complications Reduction in mortality (37.5% to 12.5%)
Rocco, 2001 [50] n = 21	Bilateral lung transplant/ ICU/PSV + PEEP		Low rate of complications and death (18/21 with no need for ETI)

Table 3. *Continued*

Author, year [ref] Number of pts	Population/ Location/Mode of ventilation	Type of study	Conclusions for NIV
Keenan, 2002 [56] n = 81	Post extubation respiratory distress	RCT	No benefit of NIV
Confalonieri, 2002 [47] n = 24	Pneumocystis carinii pneumonia	Case-control study	Improvement of ABG Reduction of ETI, of complications Reduction in mortality
Ferrer, 2002 [70] N= 105	Hypoxemic acute respiratory failure	RCT	Improvement of ABG Reduction of ETI (13 vs 29%), of septic shock Reduction in ICU mortality (18 vs 39%) and at 90 days.
Community acquired pneumonia			
Confalonieri, 1999 [40] n = 56	Community acquired pneumonia some COPD	RCT	No benefit in non COPD
Jolliet, 2001 [52] n = 24	Community acquired pneumonia	Cohort study	High intubation rate
Antonelli, 2001 [43]	Community acquired peumonia	Prospective observational study	ARDS and pneumonia: risk factors for failure
Domenighetti, 2002 [53] n = 18	Community acquired pneumonia	Cohort	Less efficacy of NIV in CAP than in pulmonary edema

trolled trials have confirmed these beneficial results ([18, 39]). As discussed later, however, patients with severe community-acquired pneumonia and hypoxemia may not represent a good indication for NIV [43].

Clinical Trials Evaluating Different Subgroups of Hypoxemic Respiratory Failure

Immunosuppression: Because one of the main benefits of NIV may be a reduction in infectious complications [44, 45], patients at high risk for nosocomial infection when mechanically ventilated may be particularly likely to benefit from NIV.

Several recent trials have shown major benefits of NIV as a preventive measure during episodes of acute hypoxemic respiratory failure in solid organ-transplant patients or in patients with severe immunosuppression, particularly related to hematological malignancies and neutropenia [38, 41, 46]. The rates of intubation and of infectious complications, length of stay, and mortality were significantly reduced by the use of NIV. Because of the high risk associated with endotracheal intubation in patients with severe immunosuppression, NIV seems to be of particular interest in this group [38, 41, 46].

Along a similar line, patients suffering from pneumocystis cariniii pneumonia during the course of human immunodeficiency virus (HIV) infection seem to benefit from NIV, as shown in a case-control study by Confalonieri et al. [47].

In immunosuppressed patients, careful selection of patients and early onset of NIV are necessary to avoid endotracheal intubation and to be beneficial to the patients.

Lung surgery: Several studies looked at the use of NIV after lung surgery [48-50]. Auriant et al. conducted a randomized controlled trial in patients who experienced respiratory distress after lung resection [49]. The reason why intubation should be avoided is the very poor outcome of patients who usually require reintubation shortly after lung surgery. A reduction in endotracheal intubation and a clear benefit in terms of hospital survival was observed with NIV. A non-controlled study suggested interesting results of using NIV in patients with respiratory distress after bilateral lung transplant [50]. NIV seems to be useful tool to prevent reintubation after lung surgery.

Community-acquired pneumonia: Confalonieri et al, in a randomized controlled trial showed major benefit of NIV in patients with community-acquired pneumonia, by reducing the number of endotracheal intubations, complications, and length of stay [40]. This benefit, however, was almost entirely explained by the subgroup of patients with COPD. The same group showed in a case-control study a benefit of NIV in patients with pneumocystis carinii pneumonia, reducing intubation, length of stay, and mortality [47]. Other studies with severely hypoxemic patients with pneumonia have shown a high rate of failure in this subgroup [43, 51-53]. More data are necessary in this group of patients and it is difficult today to recommend NIV for severe community-acquired pneumonia.

Post-extubation respiratory failure: The physiological rationale for this approach was recently demonstrated by Vitacca et al. [54]. One case-control study by Hilbert et al., suggested favorable effects of NIV to prevent reintubation in patients with COPD [55]. The prospective randomized trial by Keenan et al. was performed in all patients experiencing post-extubation respiratory distress. The study by Keenan did not find any benefit of NIV [56]. Another prospective randomized trial did not find any preventive effect of NIV [57]. In contrast, another randomized trial in COPD showed beneficial effects [58]. The question of the efficacy of NIV in preventing reintubation in all patients, therefore, remains open. The benefits of this technique may be observed only in patients with COPD.

Non-invasive Ventilation to Shorten Invasive Ventilation (Table 1)

A number of patients with COPD still require endotracheal intubation because they fail NIV, have a contraindication to NIV (such as a need for surgery), or have criteria for immediate intubation. However, when there is a need for prolonged ventilatory assistance, these patients can be switched to NIV after a few days of endotracheal intubation [59, 60]. This approach was shown to reduce the intubation time in two randomized controlled trials [59, 60]. In a study by Nava et al., complications were reduced and survival rates at day 60 were higher with this approach [59]. This benefit was not found in another study, in which the total length of ventilation was increased in the NIV arm [60]. Further studies on this potentially attractive indication for NIV are, therefore, needed.

Non-invasive Ventilation for Other Conditions

Patients not to be Intubated

Several reports have described the effects of NIV in patients with acute respiratory failure who were poor candidates for endotracheal intubation because of advanced age, debilitation, or a 'do not resuscitate' order [61, 62]. The overall success rate in these reports approximated 60 to 70 %. Gas exchange improved rapidly in successfully treated patients. Even when respiratory failure did not resolve, NIV provided symptomatic relief from dyspnea.

Patients with Acute Severe Asthma

A few studies indicate that NIV can be used in asthmatic patients [51, 63]. Two cohort studies described the beneficial short-term effects of using NIV in asthmatic patients deteriorating despite medical therapy [51, 63].

Fiberoptic Bronchoscopy

Several studies have suggested or demonstrated that fiberoptic bronchoscopy could be performed under delivery of NIV (CPAP for hypoxemic patients or pressure support + PEEP) [67–69] and that this approach improved the tolerance of bronchoscopy and could also prevent subsequent complications and need for endotracheal intubation [68].

Non-invasive Ventilation with Other Modes

Several recent studies have compared PSV to proportional assist ventilation [64-66]. The efficacy of the two techniques seemed similar, although very few patients required intubation. Studies in more severe patients are needed.

References

1. Brochard L, Isabey D, Piquet J, et al (1990) Reversal of acute exacerbations of chronic obstructive lung disease by inspiratory assistance with a face mask. N Engl J Med 323:1523-1530
2. Appendini L, Patessio A, Zanaboni S, et al (1994) Physiologic effects of positive end-expiratory pressure and mask pressure support during exacerbations of chronic obstructive pulmonary disease. Am J Respir Crit Care Med 149:1069-1076
3. Thorens JB, Ritz M, Reynard C, et al (1997) Haemodynamic and endocrinological effects of noninvasive mechanical ventilation in respiratory failure. Eur Respir J 10:2553-2559
4. Evans TW (2001) International Consensus Conferences in Intensive Care Medicine: Non-invasive positive pressure ventilation in acute respiratory failure. Intensive Care Med 27:166-178
5. Baudouin S, Blumenthal S, Cooper B, et al (2002) Non-invasive ventilation in acute respiratory failure. Thorax 57:192-211
6. Bott J, Carroll MP, Conway JH, et al (1993) Randomised controlled trial of nasal ventilation in acute ventilatory failure due to chronic obstructive airways disease. Lancet 341:1555-1557
7. Vitacca M, Rubini F, Foglio K, Scalvani S, Nava S, Ambrosino N (1993) Non invasive modalities of positive pressure ventilation improve the outcome of acute exacerbations in COLD patients. Intensive Care Med 19:450-455
8. Kramer N, Meyer TJ, Meharg J, Cece RD, Hill NS (1995) Randomized, prospective trial of noninvasive positive pressure ventilation in acute respiratory failure. Am J Respir Crit Care Med 151:1799-1806
9. Brochard L, Mancebo J, Wysocki M, et al (1995) Noninvasive ventilation for acute exacerbations of chronic obstructive pulmonary disease. N Engl J Med 333:817-822
10. Angus RM, Ahmed AA, Fenwick LJ, Peacok AJ (1996) Comparison of the acute effects on gas exchange of nasal ventilation and doxapram in acute excaerbations of chronic obstructive pulmonary disease. Thorax 51:1048-1050
11. Celikel T, Sungur M, Ceyhan B, Karakurt S (1998) Comparison of noninvasive positive pressure ventilation with standard medical therapy in hypercapnic acute respiratory failure. Chest 114:1636-1642
12. Plant PK, Owen JL, Elliott MW (2000) Early use of non-invasive ventilation for acute exacerbations of chronic obstructive pulmonary disease on general respiratory wards: a multicentre randomised controlled trial. Lancet 355:1931-1935
13. Brochard L (2000) Non-invasive ventilation for acute exacerbations of COPD : a new standard of care. Thorax 55:817-818
14. Carlucci A, Richard JC, Wysocki M, Lepage E, Brochard L, and the SRLF collaborative group on mechanical ventilation (2001) Noninvasive versus conventional mechanical ventilation. An epidemiological survey. Am J Respir Crit Care Med 163:874-880
15. Conti G, Antonelli P, Navalesi P, et al (2002) Noninvasive vs. conventional mechanical ventilation in patients with chronic obstructive pulmonary disease after failure of medical treatment in the ward: a randomized trial. Intensive Care Med 28:1701-1707
16. Vitacca M, Clini E, Rubini F, Nava S, Foglio K, Ambrosino N (1996) Non-invasive mechanical ventilation in severe chronic obstructive lung disease and acute respiratory failure: short-and long-term prognosis. Intensive Care Med 22:94-100

17. Bardi G, Pierotello R, Desideri M, Valdisseri L, Bottai M, Palla A (2000) Nasal ventilation in COPD exacerbations: early and late results of a prospective, controlled study. Eur Respir J 15:98–104
18. Confalonieri M, Parigi P, Scartabellati A, et al (1996) Noninvasive mechanical ventilation improves the immediate and long-terme outcome of COPD patients with acute respiratory failure. Eur Respir J 9:422–430
19. Corrado A, Gorini M, Ginanni R, et al (1998) Negative pressure ventilation *versus* conventional mechanical ventilation in the treatment of acute respiratory failure in COPD patients. Eur Respir J 12:519–525
20. Corrado A, Confalonieri M, Marchese S, et al (2002) Iron lung vs mask ventilation in the treatment of acute on chronic respiratory failure in COPD patients: a multicenter study. Chest 121:189–195
21. Barbé F, Togores B, Rubi M, Pons S, Maimo A, Agusti AGN (1996) Noninvasive ventilatory support does not facilitate recovery from acute respiratory failure in chronic obstructive pulmonary disease. Eur Respir J 9:1240–1245
22. Wood KA, Lewis L, Von Harz B, Kollef MH (1998) The use of noninvasive positive pressure ventilation in the emergency department: results of a randomized clinical trial. Chest 113:1339–1346
23. Jolliet P, Tassaux D, Thouret JM, Chevrolet JC (1999) Beneficial effects of helium:oxygen versus air: oxygen noninvasive pressure support in patients with decompensated chronic obstructive pulmonary disease. Crit Care Med 27:2422–2429
24. Jaber S, Fodil R, Carlucci A, et al (2000) Noninvasive ventilation with Helium-Oxygen in acute exacerbations of chronic obstructive pulmonary disease. Am J Respir Crit Care Med 161:1191–1200
25. Lin M, Yang YF, Chiang HT, Chang MS, Chiang BN, Cheitlin MD (1995) Reappraisal of continuous positive airway pressure therapy in acute cardiogenic pulmonary edema. Short-term results and long-term follow-up. Chest 107:1379–1386
26. Lenique F, Habis M, Lofaso F, Dubois-Randé JL, Harf A, Brochard L (1997) Ventilatory and hemodynamic effects of continuous positive airway pressure in left heart failure. Am J Respir Crit Care Med 155:500–505
27. L'Her E, Moriconi M, Texier F, et al (1998) Non-invasive continuous positive airway pressure in acute hypoxaemic respiratory failure—experience of an emergency department. Eur J Emerg Med 5:313–318
28. Räsänen J, Heikkilä J, Downs J, Nikki P, Vaisänen IT, Viitanen A (1985) Continuous positive airway pressure by face mask in acute cardiogenic pulmonary edema. Am J Cardiol 55:296–300
29. Bersten AD, Holt AW, Vedig AE, Skowronski GA, Baggely CJ (1991) Treatment of severe cardiogenic pulmonary edema with continuous positive airway pressure delivered by face mask. N Engl J Med 325:1825–1830
30. Masip J, Betbese AJ, Paez J, et al (2000) Non-invasive pressure support ventilation versus conventional oxygen therapy in acute cardiogenic pulmonary oedema: a randomised trial. Lancet 356:2126–2132
31. Mehta S, Gregory DJ, Woolard RH, et al (1997) Randomized, prospective trial of bilevel versus continuous positive airway pressure in acute pulmonary edema. Crit Care Med 25:620–628
32. Rusterholtz T, Kempf J, Berton C, et al (1999) Noninvasive pressure support ventilation (NIPSV) with face mask in patients with acute cardiogenic pulmonary edema (ACPE). Intensive Care Med 25:21–28
33. Hoffmann B, Welte T (1999) The use of noninvasive pressure support ventilation for severe respiratory insufficiency due to pulmonary oedema. Intensive Care Med 25:15–20
34. Sharon A, Shpirer I, Kaluski E, et al (2000) High-dose intravenous isosorbide-dinitrate is safer and better than Bi-PAP ventilation combined with conventional treatment for severe pulmonary edema. J Am Coll Cardiol 36:832–7

35. Delclaux C, L'Her E, Alberti C, et al (2000) Treatment of acute hypoxemic nohypercanic respiratory insufficiency with continuous positive airway pressure delivered by a face mask. A randomized controlled trial. JAMA 284:2352–2360
36. Wysocki M, Tric L, Wolff MA, Millet H, Herman B (1995) Noninvasive pressure support ventilation in patients with acute respiratory failure. A randomized comparison with conventional therapy. Chest 107:761–68
37. Antonelli M, Conti G, Rocco M, et al (1998) A comparison of noninvasive positive-pressure ventilation and conventional mechanical ventilation in patients with acute respiratory failure. N Engl J Med 339:429–435
38. Antonelli M, Contin G, Bufi M, et al (2000) Noninvasive ventilation for treatment of acute respiratory failure in patients undergoing solid organ transplantation. A randomized trial. JAMA 283:235–241
39. Martin TJ, Hovis JD, Costantino JP, et al (2000) A randomized, prospective evaluation of noninvasive ventilation for acute respiratory failure. Am J Respir Crit Care Med 161:807–813
40. Confalonieri M, Potena A, Carbone G, Della Porta R, Tolley EA, Meduri GU (1999) Acute respiratory failure in patients with severe community-acquired pneumonia. A prospective randomised evaluation of non-invasive ventilation. Am J Respir Crit Care Med 160:1585–1591
41. Hilbert G, Gruson D, Vargas F, et al (2001) Noninvasive ventilation in immunosuppressed patients with pulmonary infiltrates, fever, and acute respiratory failure. N Engl J Med 344:481–487
42. Rocker G, Mackenzie M, Williams B, Logan P (1999) Noninvasive positive pressure ventilation : successfull outcome in patients with acute lung injury/ARDS. Chest 115:173–177
43. Antonelli M, Conti G, Moro M, et al (2001) Predictors of failure of noninvasive positive pressure ventilation in patients with acute hypoxemic respiratory failure : a multi-center study. Intensive Care Med 27:1718–1728
44. Nourdine K, Combes P, Carton MJ, Beuret P, Cannamela A, Ducreux JC (1999) Does noninvasive ventilation reduce the ICU nosocomial infection risk? A prospective clinical survey. Intensive Care Med 25:567–573
45. Giroa E, Schortgen F, Delclaux C, et al (2000) Association of noninvasive ventilation with nosocomial infections and survival in critically III patients. JAMA 284:2361–2367
46. Azoulay E, Alberti C, Bornstain C, et al (2001) Improved survival in cancer patients requiring mechanical ventilatory support: Impact of noninvasive mechanical ventilatory support. Crit Care Med 29:519–525
47. Confalonieri M, Calderini E, Terraciano S, et al (2002) Noninvasive ventilation for treating acute respiratory failure in AIDS patients with Pneumocystis carinii pneumonia. Intensive Care Med 28:1233–1238
48. Aguilo R, Togores B, Pons S, Rubi M, Barbe F, Agusti AG (1997) Noninvasive ventilatory support after lung resectional surgery. Chest 112:117–121
49. Auriant I, Jallot A, Herve P, et al (2001) Noninvasive ventilation reduces mortality in acute respiratory failure following lung resection. Am J Respir Crit Care Med 164:1231–1235
50. Rocco M, Conti G, Antonelli M, et al (2001) Non-invasive pressure support ventilation in patients with acute respiratory failure after bilateral lung transplantation. Intensive Care Med 27:1622–1626
51. Meduri UG, Cook TR, Turner RE, Cohen M, Leeper KV (1996) Noninvasive positive pressure ventilation in status asthmaticus. Chest 110:767–774
52. Jolliet P, Abajo B, Pasquina P, Chevrolet JC (2001) Non-invasive pressure support ventilation in severe community-acquired pneumonia. Intensive Care Med 27:812–821
53. Domenighetti G, Gayer R, Gentilini R (2002) Noninvasive pressure support ventilation in non-COPD patients with acute cardiogenic pulmonary edema and severe community-acquired pneumonia : acute effects and outcome. Intensive Care Med 28:1226–1232
54. Vitacca M, Ambrosino N, Clini E, et al (2001) Physiological response to pressure support ventilation delivered before and after extubation in patients not capable of totally spontaneous autonomous breathing. Am J Respir Crit Care Med 164:638–641

55. Hilbert G, Gruson D, Portel L, Gbikpi-Benissan G, Cardinaud JP (1998) Noninvasive pressure support ventilation in COPD patients with postextubation hypercapnic respiratory insufficiency. Eur Respir J 11:1349–1353
56. Keenan S, Powers C, McCormack D, Block G (2002) Noninvasive positive-pressure ventilation for postextubation respiratory distress: a randomized controlled trial. JAMA 287:3238–3244
57. Jiang J, Kao SJ, Wang SN (1999) Effect of early application of biphasic positive airway pressure on the outcome of extubation in ventilator weaning. Respirology 4:161–165
58. Carlucci A, Gregoretti C, Squadrone V, Navalesi M, Del Mastro M, Nava S (2001) Preventive use of non-invasive mechanical ventilation to avoid post-extubation respiratory failure: a randomized controlled trial. Eur Resp J 18:29S (abst)
59. Nava S, Ambrosino N, Clini E, et al (1998) Noninvasive mechanical ventilation in the weaning of patients with respiratory failure due to chronic obstructive pulmonary disease. A randomized, controlled trial. Ann Intern Med 128:721–728
60. Girault C, Daudenthun I, Chevron V, Tamion F, Leroy J, Bonmarchand G (1999) Noninvasive ventilation as a systematic extubation and weaning technique in acute-on-chronic respiratory failure. Am J Respir Crit Care Med 160:86–92
61. Meduri GU, Fox RC, Abou-Shala N, Leeper KV, Wunderink RG (1994) Noninvasive mechanical ventilation via face mask in patients with acute respiratory failure who refused endotracheal intubation. Crit Care Med 22:1584–1590
62. Benhamou D, Girault C, Faure C, Portier F, Muir JF (1992) Nasal mask ventilation in acute respiratory failure. Experience in elderly patients. Chest 102:912–917
63. Fernandez M, Villagra A, Blanch L, Fernandez R (2001) Non-invasive mechanical ventilation in status asthmaticus. Intensive Care Med 27:486–492
64. Wysocki M, Richard J-C, Meshaka P (2002) Noninvasive proportional assist ventilation compared with noninvasive pressure support ventilation in hypercapnic acute respiratory failure. Crit Care Med 30:323–329
65. Gay P, Hess D, Hill N (2001) Noninvasive Proportional Assist Ventilation for Acute Respiratory Insufficiency. Comparison with pressure support ventilation. Am J Respir Crit Care Med 164:1606–1611
66. Patrick W, Webster K, Ludwig L, Roberts D, Wiebe P, Younes M (1996) Noninvasive positive-pressure ventilation in acute respiratory distress without prior chronic respiratory failure. Am J Respir Crit Care Med 153:1005–1011
67. Antonelli M, Conti G, Riccioni L, Meduri GU (1996) Noninvasive positive-pressure ventilation via face mask during bronchoscopy with BAL in high-risk hypoxemic patients. Chest 110:724–728
68. Maitre B, Jaber S, Maggiore S, et al (2000) Continuous positive airway pressure during fiberoptic brochoscopy in hypoxemic patients. A randomized double-blind study using a new device. Am J Respir Crit Care Med 162:1063–1067
69. Antonelli M, Conti G, Rocco M, et al (2002) Noninvasive positive-pressure ventilation vs. conventional oxygen supplementation in hypoxemic patients undergoing diagnostic bronchoscopy. Chest 121: 1149–54
70. Ferrer M, Esquinas A, Leon M, Gonzales G, Alarcon A, Torres A (2002) Non-invasive ventilation in severe acute hypoxemic respiratory failure: a randomized clinical trial. Intensive Care Med 28:S69 (abst)

Pulmonary Recruitment in Acute Lung Injury

L. Blanch, A. Villagra, and J. Lopez-Aguilar

Introduction

Mechanical ventilation is a supportive life-saving therapy in patients with acute lung injury (ALI) although it can inflict further lung damage to the lungs, indistinguishable from the pulmonary alterations attributable to ALI, if it is not appropriately applied. Several studies also suggest that mechanical ventilation can cause inflammation of the lung capable of damaging distal organs and this response can be magnified if artificial ventilation results in high intrathoracic pressure, high lung volume leading to overdistension, and cyclic alveolar recruitment and derecruitment. Two randomized controlled studies focused on studying the effects of mechanical ventilation in patients with acute respiratory distress syndrome (ARDS) have shown that the use of high tidal volumes was associated with an increase in mortality [1, 2]. In both studies, the application of a tidal volume of 6 ml/kg and a moderate or high positive end-expiratory pressure (PEEP) level increased survival. Recruitment maneuvers have been proposed as adjuncts to lung protective ventilatory strategies to forestall atelectasis when small tidal volumes and low/moderate PEEP are used in ARDS. Recruitment maneuvers are based on the assumption that almost complete alveolar recruitment could be feasible during the early course of ARDS. In this context, recruitment maneuvers could potentially recruit the lung parenchyma for gas exchange, and to prevent further lung damage to the re-aerated part of the lung.

Experimental Research on Recruitment Maneuvers

Recruitment maneuvers restored oxygenation in surfactant-depletion models of ALI. Rismensberger et al. [3] have shown in saline-lavaged rabbit lungs that a single recruitment maneuver resulted in better oxygenation without augmenting histologic injury at PEEP less than the lower inflection point (LIP) of the pressure/volume (P/V) curve, compared with the group with PEEP set above the LIP of the P/V curve without a recruitment maneuver. Furthermore, these authors, using the same model, showed that a single sustained inflation to 30 cmH_2O boosted the ventilatory cycle onto the deflation limb of the P/V curve. This strategy resulted in better oxygenation, static lung compliance and lung volumes. The different combinations of tidal volume and PEEP, and their effects on lung recruitment have an influence on the effects of recruitment maneuvers on lung function. In saline-lavaged rabbits, Bond et al. [3] showed that oxygenation improved after recruitment maneuvers during volume controlled ventilation only during low tidal ventilation (7 ml/kg) and zero end-expiratory pressure (ZEEP) and, Van der Kloot et al. [5] demonstrated no effect of recruitment maneuvers when experimental animals with ALI were ventilated with a PEEP level higher than the LIP of the static P/V curve of the respiratory system. Interestingly, Takeuchi et al. [6] demonstrated that PEEP set at 2 cmH_2O above the LIP of the P/V curve of the respiratory system was the most effective in maintaining gas exchange and minimizing lung injury compared to a PEEP level set at the maximum curvature of the deflation P/V curve. Whether recruitment maneuvers are necessary to prevent alveolar collapse over time when optimal PEEP is used remains a matter of debate. Fujino et al. [7] have shown that repetitive high-pressure recruitment maneuvers were required to maximally recruit lung in a sheep model of ARDS and, the combination of other adjuncts to mechanical ventilation can be necessary to obtain a maximal response. Cakar et al. [8] showed in an oleic acid model of ALI that recruitment maneuvers had a greater effect in the prone than supine position and the oxygenation benefit of the recruitment maneuvers was sustained in the prone position at lower PEEP compared with supine position.

Recruitment Maneuvers during Anesthesia

The rationale for using recruitment maneuvers during anesthesia is to forestall atelectasis in dependent lung areas. During anesthesia, atelectatic lung may be re-expanded by a vital capacity maneuver, or by applying an inflation pressure of 40 cmH_2O to the lungs. Re-expansion may have a sustained effect for at least 40 minutes if 40% oxygen in nitrogen is used. However, if pure oxygen is used after re-expansion, lung collapse reappears within a few minutes [9]. This time course of atelectasis suggests that gas composition and resorption phenomena play an important role in the recurrence of collapse in previously re-expanded atelectatic lung tissue.

Recruitment Maneuvers in Patients with ARDS

Lapinsky et al. [10] reported beneficial effects on oxygenation after 40 seconds of continuous PEEP of 40 cmH_2O in 14 patients with ARDS. The recruitment maneuver was considered safe although a sustained effect was achieved only if PEEP was increased after the recruitment maneuver. Using a different technique to facilitate recruitment, Pelosi et al. [11] tested the effects of periodic increases in peak airway pressure (plateau pressure of 45 cmH_2O) in patients with ARDS ventilated with PEEP (14.5 cmH_2O) and observed significant improvements in oxygenation, intrapulmonary shunt and lung mechanics. Similarly, Foti et al. [12] compared the effect of volume controlled ventilation at low PEEP with superimposition of periodic volume recruitment maneuvers with volume controlled ventilation at high PEEP in patients with ARDS. Sighs at low PEEP effectively improved oxygenation and alveolar recruitment, but were relatively less effective than a continuous high PEEP level, thus suggesting that high PEEP better stabilizes alveoli, preventing the loss in lung volume.

Two observational studies have shown a modest and variable effect of the recruitment maneuver on oxygenation when the ARDS patient is ventilated with a high level of PEEP. Richard et al. [13] demonstrated in patients with ARDS that increasing PEEP or performing a recruitment maneuver appeared to be the two strategies to counteract low tidal volume and moderate PEEP-induced de-recruitment. When recruitment maneuvers were performed in patients already ventilated with high PEEP, oxygenation modestly improved and had minimal effects on requirements for oxygenation support. Villagra et al. [14] studied the effect of a recruitment maneuver that consisted of two minutes of pressure control ventilation (mean peak airway pressure 47 ± 4.5 cmH$_2$O) and high end-expiratory pressure (mean PEEP 30 ± 4.9 cmH$_2$O) in ARDS patients receiving a lung protective approach strategy (tidal volume < 8 ml/kg and PEEP 3–4 cmH$_2$O higher than the LIP on the P/V curve). Interestingly, recruitment maneuvers did not improve oxygenation in the majority of patients regardless of the stage of ARDS, and venous admixture increased during recruitment maneuver in non-responders. This deleterious effect suggests that the recruitment maneuver increased lung volume by overdistending the more compliant already-opened and aerated alveolar units, rather than recruiting collapsed units. Alveolar overdistension would favor capillary collapse in the healthy areas and diversion of blood flow into the collapsed areas. Furthermore, a negative correlation was found between recruited lung volume induced by PEEP before recruitment maneuver and recruitment maneuver-induced changes in oxygenation. These observational studies suggest that recruitment maneuvers are not effective when the lungs have been near-optimally recruited by PEEP and tidal volume [13, 14].

Crotti et al. [15] have shown that the dynamics of recruitment and derecruitment in human ARDS of pulmonary origin are similar to those observed in oleic acid models of ALI. However, the potential for recruitment in human ARDS compared to highly recruitable animal models is rather limited. A recent study [16] found that recruitment maneuvers transiently improved oxygenation only in patients with early ARDS who did not have impairment of chest wall mechanics and with a large potential for recruitment, as was indicated by low values of lung elastance. Clearly, further studies are needed to identify with simple and reliable technology those patients who will benefit from a recruitment maneuver before recruitment maneuvers can be recommended as a routine practice to improve outcome in ARDS.

Recruitment Maneuvers after Ventilator Disconnections and during Spontaneous Breathing

Patients with ARDS need periodic suctioning of secretions due to their inability to spontaneously clear airway secretions. Lu et al. [17] studied the physiologic effects of endotracheal suctioning in anesthetized sheep and found that endotracheal suctioning was associated with atelectasis, brochoconstriction, and a decrease in arterial oxygen saturation. The combination of hyperoxygenation before the recrutiment maneuver and a recruitment maneuver after endotracheal suctioning entirely reversed the suctioning-induced increase in lung tissue resistance and atelectasis.

Diaphragmatic contraction during partial ventilatory support augments distribution of ventilation to dependent, poorly aerated but perfused lung regions. Several recent reports have suggested that the addition of periodic hyperinflations during continuous positive airway pressure (CPAP) [18], the application of sighs during pressure support ventilation (19), and the use of airway pressure release ventilation improved lung function (20). The beneficial effects of periodic sighs and spontaneous breathing seems to favor the opening of previously collapsed lung and prevent lung collapse associated with low tidal volume and low PEEP levels used in patients who are recovering from an acute episode of respiratory failure.

Conclusion

Recruitment maneuvers superimposed on mechanical ventilation have the potential to recruit atelectatic lungs in the course of general anesthesia although the physiologic benefits are less evident in patients with ARDS. Patient selection, long term benefits, and safety of recruitment maneuvers also remain to be determined. Many different methods are recommended to achieve maximal lung recruitment but no evidence exits about which should be used. Finally, evidence for the beneficial effect of recruitment maneuvers in ARDS is from non-randomized trials or from observational studies and, evidence from large, prospective and randomized clinical studies is still lacking. Therefore, the use of recruitment maneuvers in ARDS is controversial even as rescue therapy to improve oxygenation in the most severe forms of human ARDS.

References

1. Amato MBP, Barbas CSV, Medeiros DM, et al (1988) Effect of a protective-ventilation strategy on mortality in the acute respiratory distress syndrome. N Engl J Med 338:347–354
2. The Acute Respiratory Distress Syndrome Network (2000) Ventilation with lower tidal volumes as compared with traditional tidal volumes for acute lung injury and the acute respiratory distress syndrome. N Engl J Med 342:1301–1308
3. Rismensberger PC, Pristine G, Mullen JBM, et al (1999) Lung recruitment during small tidal volume ventilation allows minimal PEEP without augmenting lung injury. Crit Care Med 27:1940–1945
4. Bond JM, McAloon J, Froese AB (1994) Sustained inflations improve respiratory compliance during high-frequency oscillatory ventilation but not during large tidal volume positive pressure ventilation in rabbits. Crit Care Med 22:1269–1277
5. Van der Kloot TE, Blanch L, Youngblood AM, et al (2000) Recruitment maneuvers in three experimental models of acute lung injury. Effect of lung volume and gas exchange. Am J Respir Crit Care Med 161:1485–1494
6. Takeuchi M, Goddon S, Dolhnikoff M, et al (2002) Set positive end-expiratory pressure during protective ventilation affects lung injury. Anesthesiology 97:682–692

7. Fujino Y, Goddon S, Dolhnikoff M, Hess D, Amato MBP, Kacmarek RM (2001) Repetitive high-pressure recruitment maneuvers required to maximally recruit lung in sheep model of acute respiratory distress syndrome. Crit Care Med 29:1579–1586
8. Cakar N, Van der Kloot TE, Youngblood AM, Adams AB, Nahum A (2000) Oxygenation response to a recruitment maneuver during supine and prone positions in an oleic acid-induced lung injury model. Am J Respir Crit Care Med 161:1949–1956
9. Rothen HU, Sporre B, Enberg G, Wegenius G, Högman M, Hedenstierna G (1995) Influence of gas composition on recurrence of atelectasis after a reexpansion maneuver during general anesthesia. Anesthesiology 82:832–842
10. Lapinsky SE, Aubin M, Mehta S, Boiteau P, Slutsky AS (1999) Safety and efficacy of a sustained inflation for alveolar recruitment in adults with respiratory failure. Intensive Care Med 25:1297–1301
11. Pelosi P, Cadringher P, Bottino N, et al (1999) Sigh in acute respiratory distress syndrome. Am J Respir Crit Care Med 159:872–880
12. Foti G, Cereda M, Sparacino M, De Marchi ME, Villa F, Pesenti A (2000) Effects of periodic lung recruitment maneuvers on gas exchange and respiratory mechanics in mechanically ventilated ARDS patients. Intensive Care Med 26:501–507
13. Richard JC, Maggiore SM, Jonson B, Mancebo J, Lemaire F, Brochard L (2001) Influence of tidal volume on alveolar recruitment. Respective role of PEEP and a recruitment maneuver. Am J Respir Crit Care Med 163:1609–1613
14. Villagra A, Ochagavia A, Vatua S, et al (2002) Recruitment maneuvers during lung protective ventilation in acute respiratory distress syndrome. Am J Respir Crit Care Med 165:165–170
15. Crotti S, Mascheroni D, Caironi P, et al (2001) Recruitment and derecruitment during acute respiratory failure. A clinical study. Am J Respir Crit Care Med 164:131–140
16. Grasso S, Mascia L, Del Turco M, et al (2002) Effects of recruiting maneuvers in patients with acute respiratory distress syndrome ventilated with protective ventilatory strategy. Anesthesiology 96:795–802
17. Lu Q, Capderou A, Cluzel P, et al (2000) A computed tomographic scan assessment of endotracheal suctioning-induced bronchoconstriction in ventilated sheep. Am J Respir Crit Care Med 162:1898–1904
18. Pelosi P, Chiumallo D, Calvi E, et al (2001) Effect of different continuous positive airway pressure devices and periodic hyperinflations on respiratory function. Crit Care Med 29:1683–1689
19. Patroniti N, Foti G, Cortinovis B, et al (2002) Sigh improves gas exchange and lung volume in patients with acute respiratory distress syndrome undergoing pressure support ventilation. Anesthesiology 96:788–794
20. Putensen C, Zech S, Wrigge H, et al (2001) Long-term effects of spontaneous breathing during ventilatory support in patients with acute lung injury. Am J Respir Crit Care Med 164:43–49

Lung-Protective Ventilation Trial: A Comparison of Physiologic Effects and Patient-important Outcomes

M. O. Meade, N. Adhikari, and K. E. Burns

Introduction

Lung-protective ventilation is one of the most important advances in critical care over the past two decades. In response to a growing understanding of the lung damage that results from overdistention, cyclic alveolar collapse, and prolonged exposure to high levels of oxygen, investigators have developed and tested several ventilation strategies designed to minimize ventilator-associated lung injury.

Among the many factors that delay the implementation of results from randomized clinical trails into clinical practice, a fundamental issue is inconsistency of results among and within trials. Systematic reviews incorporating meta-analyses help to address inconsistent results among related studies. Understanding the limitations of surrogate outcomes can help clinicians to deal with apparent inconsistencies among results within single trials.

A surrogate endpoint refers to a laboratory or physiologic measurement that substitutes for a direct measurement of patient function or survival. Effects on surrogate outcomes, therefore, provide indirect evidence of benefit or harm. Surrogate outcomes are most useful when confirmation of patient-important benefit would require unduly large or long clinical trials; they are valid only when there is a strong, independent, and consistent association with a clinically important outcome.

There are many examples of discord between the effects on surrogate and patient-important outcomes, reflecting an imperfect understanding of complex physiology. For example, the antiarrhythmic agents encainide and flecainide suppress premature ventricular contractions following acute myocardial infarction and held great promise for routine care. Ultimately, they were found to increase patient mortality despite a strong physiologic rationale [1]. Similarly, a vast number of inflammatory mediator-directed therapies can reduce serum mediator levels and improve some measures of organ function among patients with sepsis; however, among more than 20 randomized controlled trials none of these agents has been found to improve survival [2]. Another notable example is that of prehospital fluid resuscitation for patients with penetrating chest trauma. Rapid improvement of hypotension is an attractive and compelling physiologic goal. However, the relatively hidden tradeoffs, hemodilution, disrupted thrombus, and increased blood loss are costly and the net effect is an iatrogenic increase in mortality [3].

The aim of this document is to highlight conflicts between physiologic outcomes and effects on survival of ventilation strategies currently used for lung-protection among patients with acute lung injury (ALI). Our aim is not to conduct a systematic review of this literature to answer questions related to inconsistent results from related trials.

Methods

We searched MEDLINE, EMBASE, CINAHL, HealthSTAR, the Cochrane Database of Systematic Reviews and the Cochrane Controlled Trials Register, from 1990 to 2002, for randomized controlled trials reporting on survival effects of 'lung-protective' strategies (tidal volume limitation, open-lung ventilation, and inhaled nitric oxide) among critically ill adults with acute lung injury (ALI). We also searched for surveys and audits of current use of these strategies in clinical practice.

Inhaled Nitric Oxide

Inhaled nitric oxide (NO), a selective pulmonary vasodilator, augments blood flow to ventilated lung units. Clinicians commonly administer inhaled NO as an adjunctive drug therapy to improve oxygenation and thereby reduce exposures to high levels of inspired oxygen and protect the lungs from ventilator-associated injury.

Four published randomized controlled trials have evaluated the effect of varying doses of inhaled NO on survival among 428 patients with ALI or acute respiratory dictress syndrome (ARDS) [4–7]. Two studies were concealed [4, 6] one was blinded [4], one included adults and children [5], and one large trial randomized only patients who were identified as "NO-responders" [6]. Cross-overs were rare, follow-up was complete, and all trials included an intention-to-treat analysis. In addition, we are aware of two industry-sponsored trials of inhaled NO therapy among approximately 600 patients with ALI or ARDS [8, 9].

Among the published trials, responses with respect to physiologic outcomes were consistent and dramatic. Inhaled NO therapy produced an acute improvement in oxygenation for, on average, 65% of patients. In two studies this translated into a sustained reduction in respiratory support [4, 5]. Effects of inhaled NO on mortality are more sobering. With one exception, all trials showed a non-statistically significant increase in mortality. The remaining study reported no effect on mortality (relative risk (RR) 0.97; 95% confidence interval [CI] 0.60-1.57) [4]. Pooling results from these four trials reveals a trend to increased mortality for patients receiving inhaled NO therapy (RR using a random effects model 1.21; 95% CI: 0.90-1.40). Although statistical aggregation of studies is controversial in the presence of clinical and statistical heterogeneity, the best current evidence suggests that inhaled NO, when applied routinely in ALI/ARDS, increases mortality.

In summary, the acute physiologic effects of inhaled NO therapy led clinicians to expect patient-important benefits, which were refuted in subsequent randomized trials. The acceptance and dissemination of this finding into routine practice contrasts with the experience of encainide and flecainide. For both interventions, physiologic responses were positive, but randomized controlled trials suggested increased mortality without a clear physiologic mechanism for harm. However, while physicians rarely use encainide and flecainide in the management of arrhythmias following acute myocardial infarction, inhaled NO is commonly used for its rapid, favorable physiologic effects.

Tidal Volume Limitation

Investigators have studied the effects of tidal volume limitation extensively in animal experiments, clinical case series and five randomized controlled trials [10–14]. The physiologic rationale is that the reduction of inspiratory pressures and volumes reduces volutrauma. However, these physiologic gains are relatively inconspicuous compared to the effects on conventional parameters of gas exchange. In fact, tidal volume limitation may worsen these physiologic outcomes, causing hypoxemia and hypercapnia. Among patients with severe ALI, marked air hunger and ventilator dyssynchrony may necessitate increased administration of sedative and neuromuscular blocking agents.

The US National Institutes of Health funded a multicenter, concealed and randomized trial of tidal volume limitation among 861 patients across the spectrum of ALI severity [10]. The two groups were similar with respect to baseline characteristics and post-randomization use of other interventions that might influence their survival. Despite the anticipated deleterious effects on gas exchange, the relative risk of hospital mortality associated with tidal volumes set at 6 ml/kg predicted body weight was 0.78 (experimental mortality rate 31.0%; control mortality 39.8%; 95% CI 0.65–0.93). This survival benefit is of the same order of magnitude as that derived from the use of aspirin in acute myocardial infarction. Though results of individual trials are not consistent in this finding, in aggregate the results of all five randomized controlled trials also suggests a clinically significant reduction in mortality. Hopefully, forthcoming systematic reviews with meta-analyses will help to clarify the reasons for different results among these related trials.

In summary, the effect of tidal volume limitation on conventional physiologic outcomes is also distinctly misleading for at least some of the low tidal volume strategies that have been tested. In contrast to the example of physiologic benefit failing to be matched by clinical benefit (inhaled NO), the observed deterioration in conventional physiologic endpoints was associated with improved survival. Nevertheless, compelling effects on physiologic parameters may play an important role in influencing clinical practice. Notwithstanding the potentially large survival advantage associated with tidal volume limitation, the findings of recent audits conducted in Asia and in North America show that the results of the NIH-sponsored trial have had limited impact on patient care [15, 16].

Open Lung Ventilation

Open lung ventilation refers to the use of strategies designed to recruit collapsed lung units for participation in gas exchange (for instance, using a lung recruitment maneuver) and to maintain ventilation among recruited lung units (with high levels of positive end-expiratory pressure [PEEP]). The goal is to ventilate within a 'safe' region of the pressure/volume (P/V) curve of the lung: applying inspiratory pressures below a level associated with regional overdistention and end-expiratory pressures above an elusive critical closing pressure [17]. The proposed mechanisms of lung protection include reductions in volutrauma, shearing injury and oxygen toxicity.

In a landmark trial comparing an open-lung strategy to a more conventional high tidal volume/low PEEP strategy, investigators enrolled 53 patients with severe ARDS and stopped the trial early in response to disproportionately high mortality in the control group [14]. They observed better oxygenation and better evolution of lung function (described as a composite measure of effects on gas exchange, lung compliance, and respiratory support) among patients in the experimental group. In this trial, favorable physiologic outcomes were mirrored by a statistically significant reduction in 28-day mortality (relative risk [RR] 0.53; 95% confidence interval [CI] 0.31-0.91).

The compelling results of this small randomized controlled trial prompted a second and larger randomized controlled trial, the 'ALVEOLI' trial, which is complete but unpublished. The investigators concealed allocation, achieved balanced cointervention use between groups and 100% follow-up, and conducted an intention-to-treat analysis. In this study, stopped prematurely in accordance with *a priori* rules for 'futility', the investigators may have missed an important benefit to the use of high PEEP.

In summary, physiologic responses to open lung ventilation are favorable but survival effects are unclear. Given the limitations of surrogate outcomes, the role for open lung ventilation will not be resolved without more data from the recently completed study and two large multicenter trials currently underway in Canada and France.

Conclusion

We have reviewed three examples of the limitations of physiologic outcomes as they relate to lung-protective ventilation trials. For two of the three interventions, basing current practice on physiologic effects may lead to iatrogenic deaths among critically ill patients with ALI.

The methods of our review included an unbiased search for relevant trials and a critical appraisal of included studies. We did not formulate or explore *a priori* hypotheses about heterogeneity among related trials; however, our aim was not to conduct a systematic review of the literature. Moreover, we did not discuss some other potentially lung-protective strategies including prone ventilation and surfactant therapy. Rather, we have presented an approach to surrogate outcomes in clinical trials of lung protection that may be useful in the face of apparently inconsistent results within trials and in the management of patients with ALI.

Based on this review, current evidence suggests that tidal volume limitation (6 ml/kg predicted body weight) is an important intervention to reduce mortality, despite the temporary worsening of gas exchange. Current evidence also suggests that clinicians should not administer inhaled NO therapy as a means of reducing oxygen toxicity, since the available evidence suggests that this may increase mortality. The results of unpublished randomized controlled trials will be extremely useful to resolve residual uncertainty on this issue. In the meantime, our findings do not apply to the use of inhaled NO for patients with severe refractory hypoxemia on 100% FiO_2 or for those patients with hemodynamically significant pulmonary hypertension. Finally, more clinical trials are needed to resolve the role for open lung ventilation in lung protection and improving survival of critically ill patients.

References

1. Echt DS, Liebson PR, Mitchell LB, et al (1991) Mortality and morbidity in patients receiving encainide, flecainide or placebo: the Cardiac Arrhythmia Suppression Trail. N Engl J Med 324:781–788
2. Eichacker PQ, Parent C, Kalil A, et al (2002) Risk and the efficacy of antiinflammatory agents. Retrospective and confirmatory studies of sepsis. Am J Respir Crit Care Med 166:1197–1205
3. Bickell WH, Wall MJ Jr, Pepe PE, et al (1994) Immediate versus delayed fluid resuscitation for hypotensive patients with penetrating torso injuries. N Engl J Med 331:1105–1109
4. Dellinger RP, Zimmerman JL, Taylor RW, et al (1998) Effects of inhaled nitric oxide in patients with acute respiratory distress syndrome: Results of a randomized phase II trial. Crit Care Med 26:15–23
5. Michael JR, Barton RG, Saffle JR, Mone M, et al (1998) Inhaled nitric oxide versus conventional therapy. Effect on oxygenation in ARDS. Am J Respir Crit Care Med 157:1372–1380
6. Lundin S, Mang H, Smithies M, Stenqvist O, Frostell C, for the European Study Group of Inhaled Nitric Oxide (1999) Intensive Care Med 25:911–919
7. Troncy E, Collet JP, Shapiro S, Guimond JG, et al (1998) Inhaled nitric oxide in acute respiratory distress syndrome. A pilot randomized controlled study. Am J Respir Crit Care Med 157:1483–1488
8. Payen D, Vallet B, and the Groupe dEtude du NO dans lARDS (1999) Results of the French prospective multicentre randomized double-blind placebo-controlled trial in inhaled nitric oxide (NO) in ARDS. Intensive Care Med 25:A645 (abst)
9. Wood KA, Linde-Zwirble WT, Clermont G, et al (2002) The effect of inhaled nitric oxide on the hospital costs of acute respiratory distress syndrome (ARDS). Am J Respir Crit Care Med 165:A220 (abst)
10. The Acute Respiratory Distress Syndrome Network (2000) Ventilation with lower tidal volumes as compared with traditional tidal volumes for acute lung injury and the acute respiratory distress syndrome. N Engl J Med 342:1301–1308
11. Brower RG, Shanholtz CB, Fessler HE, et al (1999) Prospective, randomized controlled clinical trial comparing traditional versus reduced tidal volume ventilation in acute respiratory distress syndrome patients. Crit Care Med 27:1492–1498
12. Stewart TE, Meade MO, Cook DJ, et al (1998) Evaluation of a ventilation strategy to prevent barotrauma in patients at high risk for acute respiratory distress syndrome. N Engl J Med 338:355–361

13. Brochard L, Roudot-Thoraval F, Roupie E, et al (1998) Tidal volume reduction for prevention of ventilator-induced lung injury in acute respiratory distress syndrome. The Multicenter Trail Group on Tidal Volume reduction in ARDS. Am J Respir Crit Care Med 158:1831–1838
14. Amato MB, Barbas CS, Medeiros DM, et al (1998) Effect of a protective ventilation strategy on mortality in the acute respiratory distress syndrome. N Engl J Med 338:347–54
15. Sun B, Lu Y, Zhou X, Song Z, et al (2002) A survey of adult respiratory distress syndrome in Shanghai hospitals. Am J Respir Crit Care Med 165:A218 (abst)
16. Rubenfeld GD, Caldwell E, Hudson L (2001) Publication of study results does not increase use of lung protective ventilation in patients with acute lung injury. Am J Respir Crit Care Med 163:A295 (abst)
17. Froese AB (1997) High frequency oscillatory ventilation for adult respiratory distress syndrome: lets get it right this time! Crit Care Med 25:906–908

Acute Exacerbation of Chronic Obstructive Pulmonary Diseases: What is the impact of bronchodilators, corticosteroids and antibiotics?

A. Anzueto

Introduction

Methods

Relevant articles published between 1966 and July 1st, 2002, were retrieved from Medline using the index terms "chronic obstructive pulmonary disease", "chronic bronchitis" combined with "acute exacerbations" as well as specific terms relating to various interventions such as "steroids", "bronchodilators", "anticholinergics", "antibiotics", and "mucolytics". The Cochrane control trials register until the end of the year 2001 was also searched. Well conducted, randomized, controlled trials constitute strong or *Level-A* evidence; well designed controlled trials without randomization including cohort and case control studies constitute *Level-B* or fair evidence; non-randomized clinical trials, observational studies constitute *Level-C*; and expert opinion, case studies, and before and after studies are *Level-D* or weak evidence. These ratings appear as roman numerals in parenthesis after each recommendation in these guidelines.

Epidemiology and Risk Factors

Chronic obstructive pulmonary disease (COPD) is now the 5th leading cause of death and the prevalence is increasing [1, 2]. Chronic bronchitis can be defined clinically as a disorder with expectoration of sputum on most days during at least three consecutive months for more than two successive years, other causes of cough and sputum having been excluded [3]. Chronic bronchitis accounts for approximately 85% of COPD. Chronic bronchitis frequently coexists with emphysema and small airways disease with the contribution of each disorder varying from person to person. It is essential to recognize that chronic bronchitis may occur without airway obstruction but most patients will have some evidence of COPD [4].

Acute Exacerbations of Chronic Bronchitis

Like the disease itself, exacerbations of chronic bronchitis are defined clinically. It has become traditional to use some combination of the following three criteria originally described by Anthonisen and colleagues [5] to define acute exacerbations of chronic bronchitis: increased cough and sputum, sputum purulence, and increased dyspnea over baseline. There are no validated characteristic laboratory or radiographic tests to make the diagnosis of acute exacerbations of chronic bronchitis so that definition of an exacerbation remains problematic. Seemungal and colleagues have proposed major and minor criteria to define an exacerbation. [6] The major criteria are the three proposed by Anthonisen. Minor criteria include wheeze, sore throat, cough and symptoms of a common cold such as nasal congestion or discharge. They defined an exacerbation as the presence of at least two major symptoms or one major and one minor symptom for at least two consecutive days. It is clear that the incidence of acute exacerbations of chronic bronchitis will vary depending on which definition is used. Utilizing the Anthonisen criteria the typical patient with chronic bronchitis will average 2-3 acute exacerbations of chronic bronchitis annually.

Most exacerbations, particularly those meeting the Anthonisen criteria, are believed to result from infection but exposure to allergens, pollutants or irritants (cigarette smoke, dust) may all precipitate a worsening of chronic bronchitis. Rarer causes of exacerbations include congestive heart failure, pneumonia, pulmonary emboli, pneumothorax, inappropriate oxygen administration, and drugs such as tranquilizers. Exacerbation rates are an important determinant of disease specific health status as measured by a standard quality of life questionnaire [7]. Exacerbations may lead to hospitalization which carries with it a 4% short term mortality rate for patients with mild to moderate disease [8] but as high as 24% if admitted to an intensive care unit (ICU) with respiratory failure [9-12]. This latter group of patients with severe disease have one year mortality rates of up to 46% [9-11]. Many patients requiring hospitalization for acute exacerbations of chronic bronchitis will require subsequent re-admissions because of persistent symptoms [9, 12, 13]. In addition, they will experience at least a temporary decrease in their functional abilities [14].

There are no characteristic physical findings in acute exacerbations of chronic bronchitis. Although some authors have suggested that severe exacerbations of chronic bronchitis are associated with a body temperature of >38.5 C [15] this is not widely accepted. In fact, a study of patients hospitalized because of a severe acute exacerbation of chronic bronchitis found that the mean temperature on admission was 36.4 C [9]. The presence of an elevated body temperature should suggest a viral infection [16] or underlying pneumonia as a cause of an acute exacerbation of chronic bronchitis. The lack of a clear definition of acute exacerbation of chronic bronchitis has hampered investigation into appropriate therapy of the disorder.

Chest roentgenograms are not helpful in making the diagnosis of acute exacerbation of chronic bronchitis although should be considered if there is a possibility of pneumonia or congestive heart failure contributing to the presentation. An exception to this general rule should be made for patients seen in emergency rooms or admitted to hospital. In these settings, routine chest roentgenograms have been shown to reveal abnormalities that lead to changes in management in 16–21% of patients [17–19].

Sputum Gram stain and culture have a very limited role in investigation of the etiology of acute exacerbations of chronic bronchitis since, for reasons discussed above, the airways of patients with chronic bronchitis are chronically colonized with bacteria. Therefore, the finding of a particular organism does not necessarily imply a causal relationship to the acute exacerbation of chronic bronchitis. Sputum analysis should be reserved for patients with frequent exacerbations or chronic purulent sputum in whom the presence of more virulent and/or resistant bacteria is more likely (*Level C evidence*).

Objective measurements of lung function are necessary to confirm the presence of airflow obstruction. There is a very poor correlation between chronic symptoms of dyspnea and measurement of the forced expiratory value in one second (FEV_1) [19]. In addition, there is a very poor correlation between the amount of sputum produced and the degree of airflow limitation [20, 22]. Yet the FEV_1 remains the best predictor of mortality [23] and has been shown to be important in predicting need for admission to the ICU [24]. There is also evidence that FEV_1 is highly predictive of clinical outcomes during acute exacerbations of chronic bronchitis [25]. Despite this there is continued evidence that spirometry is being underutilized in the patient group at risk of developing chronic bronchitis [26–28]. The continued reliance on clinical indicators as a basis for obtaining spirometry leads to underdiagnosis of chronic bronchitis and other causes of airflow obstruction. Despite this strong argument in favor of screening spirometry in high-risk individuals there is little evidence to suggest that spirometry has a role in evaluating an acute exacerbation of chronic bronchitis. Measurement of FEV_1 may not be possible in a patient with a severe acute exacerbation of chronic bronchitis. In addition, it is not clear that there is a correlation between transient falls in lung function and the severity of the exacerbation [6]. Therefore, although it is helpful to know the premorbid FEV_1 as a predictor of adverse outcome during an acute exacerbation of chronic bronchitis, it is not recommended that spirometry be performed during the actual exacerbation (*Level C evidence*). However, the development of an acute exacerbation of chronic bronchitis should be a motivating factor to obtain objective measurements of pulmonary function following recovery in patients who had not previously had spirometry (*Level C evidence*). The use of peak expiratory flow rates is not recommended as a substitute for spirometry as it is much more effort dependant, has not been demonstrated to predict outcome in COPD, and should not show variability in a disease defined as having fixed airflow obstruction.

Management of Acute Exacerbations of Chronic Bronchitis

Treatment of acute exacerbations of chronic bronchitis should provide symptomatic relief, prevent transient loss of pulmonary function that may lead to hospitalization, and lead to a re-evaluation of the disease in a particular patient in order to determine if the risk of future exacerbations can be reduced. Patients should be removed from any source of irritants that may worsen lower airway inflammation.

These include dust, pollutants, and first and second hand smoke. Pharmacologic therapy aims at decreasing work of breathing, reducing airway inflammation, reducing the bacterial burden in the lower airways, and treating any accompanying hypoxemia.

Bronchodilator Therapy

The majority of the studies examining the role for inhaled bronchodilators in exacerbations of COPD have been done in patients presenting to the emergency room or hospitalized because of the exacerbation. Therefore, it is not clear whether the results of these studies are applicable to the much larger population of patients with acute exacerbations of chronic bronchitis who are treated at home. In addition, the endpoint most commonly measured is FEV_1 and this may not be the most relevant parameter as it may not change much in a single acute exacerbation of chronic bronchitis. Some of the studies comparing anticholinergics to short-acting beta-agonists have combined asthmatics with COPD patients. Nonetheless, certain general statements can be made based on the available literature [29].

Most studies comparing short-acting beta-agonists to inhaled anticholinergic agents show no appreciable difference between the two in terms of effects on pulmonary function [30–33]. There may be fewer side effects with ipratropium when compared to salbutamol [34]. Most studies examining the effects of combination therapy do not report any added benefit of adding a second agent [30, 34–36]. One study demonstrated a greater improvement in FEV_1 with combination therapy compared to a beta-agonist alone [37] while another showed shorter emergency room stays for the group on combination therapy [38]. None of these studies are well standardized in terms of dose of medication or dosing frequency. Therefore, it is difficult to make specific recommendations. Some patients clearly benefit from combination bronchodilator therapy and there does not appear to be a significant increase in side effects with this combination (*Level B evidence*).

Although there has been recent interest in the role of long-acting beta-agonists in the chronic therapy of COPD these agents have not been studied in acute exacerbations of chronic bronchitis and are not recommended for treatment of this condition at the present time. A number of studies have compared the use of metered dose inhalers (MDIs) to nebulized bronchodilators. Nonetheless, as supported by a meta-analysis of studies in patients with either asthma or COPD, there does not appear to be any difference in pulmonary function outcomes between delivery systems [39]. Therefore, the choice of delivery system should be based on patient ability to use MDIs with a spacer, and cost. In most situations MDIs with an appropriate spacer would be preferred (*Level B evidence*).

There does not appear to be a role for initiation of therapy with methylxanthines in acute exacerbations of chronic bronchitis. The addition of aminophylline to inhaled bronchodilators has not been shown to lead to improved FEV_1 but does increase side effects [40, 41]. For patients who are already on an oral methylxanthine product it is reasonable to continue the medication during an acute exacerbation. However, one must keep in mind possible drug interactions with antibiotics (e.g., ciprofloxacin, clarithromycin) and adjust the dose accordingly (*Level C evidence*).

Corticosteroid Therapy

A number of randomized, placebo-controlled trials have been published confirming the value of oral and/or parenteral corticosteroids in the therapy of acute exacerbations of chronic bronchitis. These trials are summarized in Table 1. These studies definitively demonstrate that systemic steroids lead to a faster improvement in pre- and post-bronchodilator FEV1, more rapid recovery of PaO_2, decreased treatment failures and shorter hospitalization rates. One other randomized, placebo-controlled trial revealed similar benefits of hydrocortisone 100 mg IV every 4 hours for 4 days followed by 40 mg of prednisone daily for another 4 days [42]. This study is not included in the table because it is not clear that asthmatics were excluded from the trial. In addition, the attending physicians were allowed to add hydrocortisone 100 mg IV every 4h in addition to the study drug if they believed the patient must have steroids. This led to a change in therapy for 12 out of 87 patients admitted to hospital. The one negative study failing to show a benefit of parenteral steroids during an exacerbation of COPD used only a single dose of methylprednisolone 100 mg in the emergency room and measured FEV_1 outcomes 1 and 3 hours following this bolus [43]. Therefore, the follow-up interval may not have been sufficient to detect a significant improvement as it is generally felt that steroids take at least 6 hours to have a beneficial effect.

There are a number of limitations to these trials. All but one of the studies [44] were performed in emergency rooms or hospital wards so that the results may not be applicable to outpatient populations. The severity of the underlying lung disease was quite variable although the majority of patients enrolled had moderate to severe underlying disease. Finally, the dose and duration of corticosteroid therapy varied widely among studies making it virtually impossible to provide specific treatment recommendations. One must carefully weigh the pros and cons of higher doses and more prolonged corticosteroid therapy in this elderly group of individuals. In the studies quoted, the major side effect in the steroid treated group was hyperglycemia [45, 46].

Systemic therapy may have additional beneficial effects aside from speeding up recovery from an acute exacerbation of chronic bronchitis. A retrospective study performed in an emergency room setting demonstrated that steroid treated individuals had a significantly reduced likelihood of relapse compared to the group not getting steroids [47]. Seemungal and colleagues followed a cohort of 101 COPD outpatients over 2.5 years during which a total of 504 exacerbations were recorded. It was up to the individual treating physician to choose whether or not to add steroids to the treatment plan for any patient [6]. Patients receiving prednisolone had more severe exacerbations as reflected by larger falls in peak expiratory flow rate and a longer recovery time for symptoms and peak expiratory flow rate. However, the rate of recovery of peak expiratory flow rate was faster in the group given prednisolone. Of greater interest, steroids greatly prolonged the time to the next exacerbation from a median of 60 days in the group not receiving prednisolone to 84 days in the treated group (p=0.037). In contrast, antibiotic therapy had no effect on recovery time or time to next exacerbation.

There is good evidence to support the use of oral or parenteral steroids for most moderate to severe patients with acute exacerbations of chronic bronchitis (*Level A evidence*). The exact dose and duration of therapy should be individualized and more specific recommendations must await further evidence. It appears that 10 days of therapy is more effective than 3 days but no other comparisons have been made [48]. We recommend treatment for periods of less than 14 days (*Level-IC evidence*). Whether patients with mild disease ($FEV_1 \geq 60$–70% predicted) also benefit from a course of oral steroids during acute exacerbations of chronic bronchitis is unknown at the present time. There are significant health consequences to the use of continuous oral corticosteroids in COPD and similar deleterious effects may occur in patients treated with frequents short courses [49].

The role for inhaled steroids in acute exacerbations of chronic bronchitis has not yet been defined. Although some studies have failed to demonstrate a role for inhaled steroids in speeding up symptom resolution in acute exacerbations of chronic bronchitis, these trials have not been designed to answer this question [50]. A recently published prospective, randomized trial comparing high dose nebulized budesonide (2 mg 6 hrly for 72 hrs) versus prednisone (30 mg twice daily for 72 hrs), demonstrated no difference between active treatments, with both being superior to placebo in terms of recovery of FEV_1 [51].

Antibiotic Therapy

Despite many decades of therapeutic trials, the role for antimicrobial therapy in acute exacerbations of chronic bronchitis remains controversial. There are a number of reasons for this. Most comparative antimicrobial trials demonstrate equivalence [1]. These trials are mainly performed for registration purposes. Accordingly, they are powered to demonstrate equivalence only as required by the licensing authorities, and intrinsic superiority such as improved in-vitro activity or excellent pharmacokinetics and/or pharmacodynamics cannot be demonstrated. Complicated patients with pre-treatment resistant pathogens or with co-morbid conditions that might interfere with the activity or assessment of the antimicrobial are usually systematically excluded. Most clinical studies do not capture subtle outcome differences between agents such as speed of recovery, microbiological eradication rates, and time to next occurrence. As currently designed, these studies demonstrate the efficacy of the antimicrobial but cannot demonstrate effectiveness (performance in real life circumstances). This part of the document will emphasize data supporting the use of antibiotics in acute exacerbations of chronic bronchitis. Emerging concepts regarding antimicrobial resistance will be discussed.

The controversial role of antibiotics has been somewhat clarified by recent studies. Randomized, placebo-controlled antimicrobial trials conducted in previous decades were inconclusive [52–57] (Table 2). Many of the earlier studies were not powered to reach a definitive conclusion but more recent well-designed studies

Table 1. Randomized trials of corticosteroids in COPD exacerbations

Study [Ref]	Year	Sample Size	Intervention	Outcomes	p-value Steroids vs. Placebo
Emerman [43]	1989	96	methylprednisolone 100 mg × 1	FEV1 at 3 and 5 hours Admission	NS NS
Albert [104]	1980	44	methylprednisolone 0.5 mg/kg q6h × 72 hrs	pre- and post-bronchodilator FEV1 tid × 72 hrs	p<0.001
Thompson [44]	1996	27	prednisone 30 mg × 3 days, 40 mg × 3 days, 20 mg × 3 days	improvement in PO_2 improvement FEV1 decreased treatment failures	p=0.002 p=0.006 p=0.002
Davies [45]	1999	56	prednisolone 30 mg od × 2 weeks	FEV_1 post-bronchodilator length of hospitalization	p<0.0001 p=0.027
Niewoehner [46]	1999	271	methylprednisolone 125 mg q6h × 72 hrs followed by prednisone 60 mg od × 4 days tapered over 2 versus 6 weeks	treatment failure length of hospitalization increased FEV_1 days 1–3	p=0.04 p=0.03 p<0.05
Maltais [51]	2002	199	prednisolone 30 mg q12h × 6 budesonide 2mg q6h × 3 days	post-bronchodilator FEV1	p<0.05 v placebo NS BUD vs pred

have concluded that antibiotics are effective. Anthonisen and coworkers, in a landmark study, developed a classification system to identify patients likely to be infected with bacterial pathogens based upon presenting clinical symptoms [5]. A type I exacerbation is defined as a patient presenting with increased dyspnea, increased sputum volume, and sputum purulence. A type II exacerbation refers to a patient with two of these symptoms, while a type III exacerbation occurs when a patient has only one symptom. Patients exhibiting a type I or type II exacerbation have a demonstrable benefit from antimicrobial therapy (more likely to resolve in 21 days, more rapid recovery of peak flow, shorter clinical illness, fewer patients exhibiting deterioration after the first 72 hours) implying a bacterial etiology, while those with a type III exacerbation do not differ from patients receiving placebo. Allegra and co-workers in another well-designed, randomized trial involving a large number of patients, demonstrated the superiority of amoxicillin/clavulanate to placebo [58]. A more recent randomized, double-blind, placebo-controlled study in 93 mechanically ventilated patients with an exacerbation demonstrated that the use of fluoroquinolones compared to placebo was associated with a reduction in mortality, duration of hospital stay and time on mechanical ventila-

Table 2. Randomized trials of antibiotics in acute exacerbations of chronic bronchitis

Comparisons	No. of Patients	Outcome of Therapy	Reference
Placebo v.	37	treated patients lost half as much time from work and exacerbations were shorter	Elmes et al 1957 [52]
Oxytetracycline	37		
Placebo v.	27	treated patients recovered sooner and deteriorated less often	Berry et al 1960 [53]
Oxytetracycline	26		
Placebo v.	28	no significant difference in clinical response	Elmes et al 1965 [54]
Ampicillin	28		
Placebo v.	10	no significant differences	Peterson et al 1967 [55]
physiotherapy v.	10		
chloramphenicol	9		
Placebo v.	86	antibiotic therapy superior to placebo but no differences between antibiotics	Pines et al 1972 [56]
chloramphenicol	84		
v. tetracycline	89		
Placebo v.	20	100% vs. 100% clinical response	Nicotra et al 1982 [57]
Tetracycline	20		
Placebo v. either co-trimoxazole, amoxicillin or doxycycline	180 182	55% versus 68% success ($p<0.01$)	Anthonisen et al 1987 [5]
Placebo v.	179	50.3% vs	Allegre et al 1991 [58]
co-amoxiclav	190	86.4% success ($p<0.01$)	
Placebo v.	47	Absolute risk reduction of 45.9 in death or need for additional antibiotics in ventilated patients ($p<0.0001$)	Nouira et al 2001 [59]
Ofloxacin	46		

tion, and a decrease in the need for additional antibiotics [59]. A conflicting study purporting to show no benefit of antibiotic therapy is flawed by including patients with relatively mild disease and/or asthma with the latter group undoubtedly improving due to the oral steroids that the patients were given [60].

Although the Anthonisen classification is helpful in predicting an antimicrobial response, it has only a sensitivity of 59% and specificity of 60% in predicting a bacterial exacerbation [61]. While an advance, this would suggest that this particular classification system is only moderately successful in predicting a bacterial etiology and confirming the role of antimicrobials. The presence of green (purulent) secretions in a patient with a history of COPD is 99.4% sensitive and 77.0%

specific for the yield of high bacterial load and may identify a clear subset of patients likely to benefit from antibiotic therapy [62]. It should be pointed out that the patients in this study all had increased dyspnea, so that they were all at least Anthonisen Type II. In a meta-analysis examining placebo-controlled trials in acute exacerbations of chronic bronchitis, antibiotic therapy improved clinical outcomes and hastened clinical and physiological recovery [63].

Traditionally, older antibiotics such as ampicillin, tetracycline or trimethoprim/sulfamethoxazole, have been the standard treatment choices for acute exacerbations of chronic bronchitis. The development of resistance of primary respiratory pathogens to these antibiotics, the recognition of more virulent Gram-negative organisms especially among patients with significant impairment of lung function, and the development of more potent, broad spectrum agents with improved coverage of the major respiratory pathogens has forced a re-examination of antimicrobial choices.

A failure rate that varies from 13–25% can be expected after treatment with traditional first line antibiotics (amoxicillin, trimethoprim/sulphamethoxazole, tetracycline, erythromycin) [64–66]. This initial treatment failure can be associated with enormous additional expenditures especially among patients with significant compromise of lung function. These patients tend to require hospitalization and are at risk for the development of respiratory failure [66]. Resistance to β-lactam antibiotics such as ampicillin can be expected in 40% of isolated strains of *Haemophilus influenzae* and in greater than 90% of strains of *Moraxella catarrhalis* [67, 68]. There are no clinical features that can predict the presence of β-lactamase producing bacteria except that patients with these organisms tend to have more courses of antibiotics [69]. Penicillin resistance is now found in > 35% of *Streptococcus pneumoniae* isolates in some studies and is increasing worldwide [70]. Penicillin resistance in Canada has been reported to be as high as 30% [71]. Penicillin resistance is also a marker for resistance to other classes of antibiotics including the cephalosporins, macrolides, β-lactam/β-lactamase inhibitors, trimethoprim-sulfamethoxazole, and tetracyclines [72]. Whereas antibiotic resistance and widespread clinical failure in lower respiratory tract infections have not been linked at this time, this may only be a reflection of the rapidly changing antimicrobial environment. Most organisms demonstrate low levels of penicillin resistance (minimal inhibitory concentration [MIC] ≤ 2 g/ml). Since the doses of β-lactams usually prescribed achieve high levels in blood, these current levels of resistance may be overcome. If levels of resistance continue to increase, however, the value of many classes of antibiotics including β-lactams, cephalosporins, macrolides, tetracyclines, and trimethoprim-sulfonomide combinations may diminish. Antibiotic overprescribing for non bacterial infections is a major factor in the emergence of bacterial resistance. Attention must be paid to improving antibiotic use as well as to identifying those patients who would benefit from aggressive broad-spectrum therapy. One advantage of a risk stratification system is that patients not requiring antimicrobial therapy can be identified as well as those requiring more aggressive therapy.

Summary of Evidence Regarding Antibiotic Therapy for Acute Exacerbations of Chronic Bronchitis (Table 3)

1. Antimicrobial therapy is warranted for patients with an acute exacerbation of chronic bronchitis if they fall into the Anthonisen type I or type II categories (*Level A evidence*, 2 randomized, large scale double-blind trials, 1 meta-analysis)
2. Antimicrobial therapy is not warranted for patients with a type III exacerbation (*Level A evidence*).
3. Patients can be stratified according to their risk of treatment failure (*Level C, D evidence*)
4. A high-risk group of patients can be identified on clinical grounds and the major clinical features are significant impairment of lung function (FEV_1 ≤50% predicted), frequent exacerbations (≥ 4/year), long duration of disease, significant co-morbidity, advanced age, malnutrition, and chronic oral corticosteroid use. (*Level C evidence*)
5. Risk group 0 patients (acute tracheobronchitis) should not be treated with antibiotics unless symptoms persist beyond 7 to 10 days (*Level A evidence*)
6. For risk group 0 patients with persistent symptoms, a macrolide or tetracycline is recommended since *Mycoplasma pneumoniae*, *Chlamydia pneumoniae*, or *Bordetella pertussis* may be pathogens (*LevelC evidence*)
7. Although resistant *H. influenzae* and *M. catarrhalis* may be pathogens, traditional first-line agents (aminopenicillins, doxycycline, trimethaprim-sulphamethoxazole) continue to be efficacious and are recommended for patients without risk factors for treatment failure (*Level B evidence*). Second generation macrolides and some second and third generation cephalosporins (cefuroxine, cefprozil, cefixime) may be better choices given concerns regarding emerging antimicrobial resistance (*Level C evidence*).
8. There are no data to demonstrate that, among Group I patients (low risk for treatment failure), that there is any clinical or economic benefit derived from using more potent, broader spectrum agents (*Level A evidence*).
9. Broad-spectrum potent agents such as fluoroquinolones or amoxicillin/clavulanate are recommended for group II patients (*Level C evidence*).
10. There is some evidence that fluoroquinolones perform better than other agents for group II patients (*Level B evidence*)
11. Group III patients at risk for *Pseudomonas aeruginosa* infection (frequent antimicrobials, structural lung damage, and chronic corticosteroids) should be treated with an anti-pseudomonal agent (ciprofloxacin). Alternative agents currently must be given parenterally (*Level C evidence*).
12. Patients presenting with a relapse or recurrence of acute exacerbation of chronic bronchitis, within 3 months of previous antibiotic therapy, should be treated with a different class of antibiotics (*Level C evidence*)

Table 3. Risk classification and suggested antimicrobial therapy [1, 3]

Group	Basic Clinical State	Symptoms and Risk Factors	Probable Pathogens	First Choice	Alternatives for Treatment Failure
0	Acute tracheo-bronchitis	Cough & sputum without previous pulmonary disease	Usually viral	None unless symptoms persist for > 7 to 10 days	Macrolide or tetracycline
I	Chronic bronchitis without risk factors (Simple)	Increased cough and sputum, sputum purulence, and increased dyspnea	H. influenzae, Haemophilus spp., M. catarrhalis, S. pneumoniae Amoxicillin, doxycycline, trimethoprim/sulphamethoxazole	Second generation macrolide, second or third generation cephalosporin, inhibitor	Fluoro-quinolone, β-lactam/β-lactamase
II	Chronic bronchitis with risk factors (Complicated)	As in class I plus (at least one of): • FEV1<50% predicted • ≥ 4 exacerbations/year • Age > 65 years • Significant co-morbidity (especially heart disease) • Use of home oxygen • Chronic oral steroid use • Antibiotic use in the past 3 months	As in class I plus • Klebsiella spp. + other Gram-negatives • Increased probability of β-lactam resistance	Fluoroquinolone, β-lactam/β-lactamase inhibitor	may require parenteral therapy consider referral to a specialist or hospital
III	Chronic suppurative bronchitis	• As in class II with constant purulent sputum; • Some have bronchiectasis • FEV1, usually < 35% predicted or • Multiple risk factors (e.g. frequent exacerbations and FEV1 <50%	As in class II plus *Pseudomonas aeruginosa* and multi-resistant Enterobacteriaciae	Ambulatory patients: tailor treatment to airway pathogen *P. aeruginosa* common (ciprofloxacin); Hospitalized patients: parenteral therapy usually required.	

Miscellaneous Therapies

At this point there is no evidence supporting the use of leukotriene (LT) receptor antagonists (LTRAs) in acute exacerbations of chronic bronchitis. These agents block the actions of the cysteinyl leukotrienes that have an important role in asthma but no demonstrable effect in COPD. The currently available LTRAs have no effect on LTB4, which does have a role in the pathogenesis of chronic bronchitis and acute exacerbations of chronic bronchitis. Future studies will examine the effects of specific LTB4 antagonists in acute exacerbations of chronic bronchitis.

The use of non-invasive ventilation (NIV) in acute exacerbations of COPD has been demonstrated to reduce mortality and decrease the need for intubation and mechanical ventilation [73, 74](*Level A evidence*). Overall, NIV also reduces morbidity and hospital or ICU length of stay [75]. Factors predicting success include good level of consciousness at the start of the trial, higher pH and lower $PaCO_2$, and improvements in pH and $PaCO_2$ within 1 hour of NIV initiation [76–78]. Poor outcomes are associated with decreased adherence to NIV protocol, presence of pneumonia and poor nutritional status.

Prevention of Acute Exacerbations of Chronic Bronchitis

Cigarette smoking remains the primary risk factor for the development of chronic bronchitis. Although only 15% of smokers will develop airflow obstruction, more than half will develop chronic cough and sputum production with subsequent increased risk for bacterial colonization and recurrent episodes of acute exacerbation of chronic bronchitis. Unfortunately, in 1999, there were slightly more than 6 million smokers in Canada representing 25% of the population age 15 and older [79]. Any intervention that slows the rate of decline in FEV_1 is likely to have a major impact on survival in patients with chronic bronchitis. Smoking cessation has clearly been shown to reduce the rate of decline of FEV_1 [79]. The benefits in terms of decline of lung function are seen even in those over the age of 60 [80]. In addition, cessation of smoking has been shown to confer a survival advantage (*Level B evidence*) [81]. Smoking cessation leads to dramatic symptomatic benefits for patients with chronic bronchitis (*Level C evidence*). Coughing stops in as many as 77% of patients who quit smoking and improves in another 17%. When coughing stops, it does so within 4 weeks in 54% of patients [82]. Evidence is lacking that this decrease in cough and sputum production will lead to a subsequent decline in the frequency of acute exacerbations of chronic bronchitis. It is known that patients with chronic cough and sputum production have increased acute exacerbation episodes compared to similarly matched smoking control patients so that the hope is that smoking cessation will lead to fewer exacerbations. Nonetheless, this enthusiasm must be tempered by the fact that there is evidence for ongoing airway inflammation even in patients with COPD who do not currently smoke [83, 84]. A recent analysis of patients in the Lung Health Study revealed that recurrent lower respiratory infections hastened the decline in FEV_1 in current smokers but not-ex-smokers [85].

A detailed discussion of smoking cessation can be found elsewhere [86]. No single technique to encourage smoking cessation is successful in all groups of patients; however, recent studies using a combination of behavioral counselling, nicotine replacement and pharmacologic therapy to decrease the desire to smoke revealed one year abstinence rates of as high as 35.5% [87]. A discussion of smoking behavior and the setting of a specific cessation date should be part of every physician-patient encounter (*Level C evidence*).

Patients with chronic lung disease have a higher risk for complications from influenza infection. By virtue of its ability to further damage airway epithelial cells influenza infection can lead to secondary bacterial proliferation and an increase in the frequency of acute exacerbations of chronic bronchitis. Serological evidence of influenza A or B infection has been found in up to 28% of patients with acute exacerbations of chronic bronchitis [87, 88, 90]. In addition, COPD patients infected with influenza have a significant risk of requiring hospitalization [91]. Perhaps this is related to the transient decline in pulmonary function caused by influenza in a group of patients with less pulmonary reserve [92]. Annual influenza vaccination reduces morbidity and mortality of influenza in the elderly by 50%. In addition, it reduced the incidence of hospitalization for acute and chronic respiratory conditions by as much as 39%[93, 94]. Therefore, the use of an annual influenza vaccine for all patients with chronic bronchitis is strongly recommended (*Level B evidence*). The role for either oral or inhaled neuraminidase inhibitors which are effective against strains of both influenza A and B is currently being studied in terms of preventing AECB during influenza outbreaks in high-risk patients. Therefore, no current evidence-based recommendations can be made. However, high risk patients who have not been vaccinated should receive prophylaxis during an outbreak (*Level C evidence*).

The value of pneumococcal vaccination in patients with chronic bronchitis is less well established. At least two meta-analyses looking at efficacy of a 17-valent or less vaccine resulted in opposite conclusions [95, 96]. Since 1983, a 23-valent vaccine has been available and this covers 85% of the serotypes responsible for invasive pneumococcal infection. Use of this vaccine in elderly patients with chronic lung disease revealed a significant lower risk for pneumonia, hospitalization and death, and direct medical care cost savings [97]. However, acute exacerbation of chronic bronchitis is a mucosal infection and it is unclear whether or not this vaccine can reduce the incidence of this complication of chronic bronchitis. Some reports state that the vaccine has up to a 65% efficacy in patients with COPD but do not specifically comment on acute exacerbations of chronic bronchitis [98]. It is generally agreed that pneumococcal vaccination is safe and can reduce invasive pneumococcal infection leading to current recommendations for vaccinations in all patients with COPD at least once in their lives. In addition, consideration should be given to repeating the vaccine in 5 to 10 years in high-risk patients [99] (*Level C evidence*).

A meta-analysis published in 1998 suggested that oral mucolytic agents such as N-acetylcysteine or iodinated glycerol reduced the frequency of acute exacerbations of chronic bronchitis, disability days, and antibiotic use [100]. The greatest effects were seen in patients who had a large number of exacerbations. Oral mucolytic agents reduced exacerbations by 22% in patients who had an average of

5.5 exacerbations per year. However, a more typical chronic bronchitic patient with 2 to 3 exacerbations per year would expect to reduce exacerbations by less than 1 by taking mucolytic agents daily for 2 to 3 years. No effect on rate of decline of FEV_1 was seen. A more recent meta-analysis on the effect of oral N-acetylcysteine revealed similar results in terms of a decrease in acute exacerbations of chronic bronchitis in patients treated for 12–24 weeks [101]. In addition, a recently published update of Poole's Cochrane analysis confirmed the beneficial results of N-acetylcysteine and determined that the number of patients needed to treat for one patient to have no exacerbations during the study period was 6 [102]. A study in Switzerland suggested that therapy with N-acetylcysteine was cost effective [103]. The mechanism by which N-acetylcysteine reduces acute exacerbations of chronic bronchitis is unclear but may be related to enhancing macrophage activity which would help defend against mucosal infections [104]. N-acetylcysteine therapy should be considered in patients with more than 5 exacerbations per year (*Level A evidence*).

References

1. Balter M, Hyland R, Low D (1994) Recommendations on the management of chronic bronchitis: A practical guide for Canadian physicians. Can Med Assoc J 151(Suppl):7–33
2. Mannino DM, Homa DM, Akinbani LJ, Ford E, Redd SC (2000) Chronic Obstructive Pulmonary Disease Surveillance United States, 1971–2000. MMWR Surveill Summ 51:1–16
3. Snow S, Lascher S, Mottur-Pilson C for the Joint Expert Panel on Chronic Obstructive Pulmonary Disease of the ACCP and the ACP-ASIM (2001) Evidence base for management of acute exacerbation of chronic obstructive pulmonary disease. Ann Intern Med 134:595–599
4. Oswald NC, Harold JT, Martin WJ (1953) Clinical pattern of chronic bronchitis. Lancet 2:693–743
5. Anthonisen NR, Manfreda J, Warren CP, Hershfield ES, Harding GK, Nelson NA (1987) Antibiotic therapy in exacerbations of chronic obstructive pulmonary disease. Ann Intern Med 106:196–204
6. Seemungal TA, Donaldson GC, Bhowmik A, Jeffries DJ, Wedzicha JA (2000) Time course and recovery of exacerbations in patients with chronic obstructive pulmonary disease. Am J Respir Crit Care Med 161:1608–1613
7. Seemungal TA, Donaldson GC, Paul EA, Bestall JC, Jeffries DJ, Wedzicha JA (1998) Effect of exacerbation on quality of life in patients with chronic obstructive pulmonary disease. Am J Respir Crit Care Med 157 (5:Pt 1):1418–1422
8. Mushlin AI, Black ER, Connolly CA, Buonaccorso KM, Eberly SW (1991) The necessary length of hospital stay for chronic pulmonary disease. JAMA 266:80–83
9. Connors AF, Dawson NV, Thomas C, et al (1996) Outcomes following acute exacerbation of severe chronic obstructive lung disease. The SUPPORT investigators (Study to Understand Prognoses and Preferences for Outcomes and Risks of Treatments). Am J Respir Crit Care Med 154 (4:Pt 1):959–967
10. Burk RH, George RB (1973) Acute respiratory failure in chronic obstructive pulmonary disease. Immediate and long-term prognosis. Arch Intern Med 132:865–868
11. Seneff MG, Wagner DP, Wagner RP, Zimmerman JE, Knaus WA (1995) Hospital and 1-year survival of patients admitted to intensive care units with acute exacerbation of chronic obstructive pulmonary disease. JAMA 274:1852–1857
12. Cydulka RK, McFadden ER Jr, Emerman CL, Sivinski LD, Pisanelli W, Rimm AA (1997) Patterns of hospitalization in elderly patients with asthma and chronic obstructive pulmonary disease. Am J Respir Crit Care Med 156:1807–1812

13. Osman IM, Godden DJ, Friend JA, Legge JS, Douglas JG (1997) Quality of life and hospital re-admission in patients with chronic obstructive pulmonary disease. Thorax 52:67–71
14. Peach H, Pathy MS (1981) Follow-up study of disability among elderly patients discharged from hospital with exacerbations of chronic bronchitis. Thorax 36:585–589
15. Hagedorn SD (1992) Acute exacerbations of COPD. How to evaluate severity and treat the underlying cause. Postgrad Med 91:105–107
16. Seemungal T, Harper-Owen R, Bhowmik A, et al (2001) Respiratory viruses, symptoms, and inflammatory markers in acute exacerbations and stable chronic obstructive pulmonary disease. Am J Respir Crit Care Med 164:1618–23
17. Emerman CL, Cydulka RK (1993) Evaluation of high-yield criteria for chest radiography in acute exacerbation of chronic obstructive pulmonary disease. Ann Emerg Med 22:680–684
18. Tsai TW, Gallagher EJ, Lombardi G, Gennis P, Carter W (1993) Guidelines for the selective ordering of admission chest radiography in adult obstructive airway disease. Ann Emerg Med 22:1854–1858
19. Sherman S, Skoney JA, Ravikrishnan KP (1989) Routine chest radiographs in exacerbations of chronic obstructive pulmonary disease. Diagnostic value. Arch Intern Med 149:2493–2496
20. Jamal K, Cooney TP, Fleetham JA, Thurlbeck WM (1984) Chronic bronchitis. Correlation of morphologic findings to sputum production and flow rates. Am Rev Respir Dis 129:719–722
21. Wolkove N, Dajczman E, Colacone A, Kreisman H (1989) The relationship between pulmonary function and dyspnea in obstructive lung disease. Chest 96:1247–1251
22. Peto R, Speizer F, Cochrane A, et al (1983) The relevance in adults of air-flow obstruction but not of mucus hypersecretion, to morality from chronic lung disease. Results from 20 years of prospective observation. Am Rev Respir Dis 128:491–500
23. Hodgkin JE (1990) Prognosis in chronic obstructive pulmonary disease. Clin Chest Med 11:555–569
24. Vitacca M, Clini E, Porta R, Foglio K, Ambrosino N (1996) Acute exacerbations in patients with COPD: predictors of need for mechanical ventilation. Eur Respir J 9:1487–1493
25. Niewoehner D, Collins D, Erbland M (2000) Relation to FEV1 to clinical outcomes during exacerbations of chronic obstructive pulmonary disease. The Department of Veterans Affairs Cooperative Study Group. Am J Respir Crit Care Med 161:1201–1205
26. Mannino DM, Etzel RA, Flanders WD (1993) Do the medical history and physical examination predict low lung function? Arch Intern Med 153:1892–1897
27. Kesten S, Chapman K (1993) Physician perceptions and management of COPD. Chest 104:254–258
28. Renwick DS, Connolly MJ (1996) Prevalence and treatment of chronic airways obstruction in adults over the age of 45. Thorax 51:164–168
29. Kuhl DA, Agiri OA, Mauro LS (1994) Beta-agonists in the treatment of acute exacerbation of chronic obstructive pulmonary disease. Ann Pharmacother 28:1379–1388
30. Emerman CL, Cydulka RK (1997) Effect of different albuterol dosing regimens in the treatment of acute exacerbation of chronic obstructive pulmonary disease. Ann Emerg Med 29:474–478
31. ODriscoll BR, Taylor RJ, Horsley MG, Chambers DK, Bernstein A (1989) Nebulised salbutamol with and without ipratropium bromide in acute airflow obstruction. Lancet 1:1418–1420
32. Backman R, Helstrom P (1985) Fenoterol and ipratropium bromid for treatment of patients with chronic bronchitis. Curr Ther Res 38:135–140
33. Karpel JP, Pesin J, Greenberg D, Gentry E (1990) A comparison of the effects of ipratropium bromide and metaproterenol sulfate in acute exacerbations of COPD. Chest 98:835–839
34. Rebuck AS, Chapman KR, Abboud R, et al (1987) Nebulized anticholinergic and sympathomimetic treatment of asthma and chronic obstructive airways disease in the emergency room. Am J Med 82:59–64
35. Moayyedi P, Congleton J, Page RL, Pearson SB, Muers MF (1995) Comparison of nebulised salbutamol and ipratropium bromide with salbutamol alone in the treatment of chronic obstructive pulmonary disease. Thorax 50:834–837

36. Patrick DM, Dales RE, Stark RM, Laliberte G, Dickinson G (1990) Severe exacerbations of COPD and asthma. Incremental benefit of adding ipratropium to usual therapy. Chest 98:295–297
37. Cydulka RK, Emerman CL (1995) Effects of combined treatment with glycopyrrolate and albuterol in acute exacerbation of chronic obstructive pulmonary disease. Ann Emerg Med 25:470–473
38. Shrestha M, OBrien T, Haddox R, Gourlay HS, Reed G (1991) Decreased duration of emergency department treatment of chronic obstructive pulmonary disease exacerbations with the addition of ipratropium bromide to beta-agonist therapy. Ann Emerg Med 20:1206–1209
39. Turner M, Patel A, Ginsburg S, FitzGerald J (1997) Bronchodilator delivery in acute airflow obstruction. A meta-analysis. Arch Intern Med 157:1736–1744
40. Rice KL, Leatherman JW, Duane PG, et al (1987) Aminophylline for acute exacerbations of chronic obstructive pulmonary disease. A controlled trial. Ann Intern Med 107:305–309
41. Seidenfeld JJ, Jones WN, Moss RE, Tremper J (1984) Intravenous aminophylline in the treatment of acute bronchospastic exacerbations of chronic obstructive pulmonary disease. Ann Emerg Med 13:248–252
42. Bullard M, Liaw S, Tsai Y, Min H (1996) Early corticosteroid use in acute exacerbations of chronic airflow obstruction. Am J Emerg Med 14:139–143
43. Emerman C, Connors A, Lukens T, May M, Effron D (1989) A randomized controlled trial of methylprednisolone in the emergency treatment of acute exacerbations of COPD. Chest 95:563–567
44. Thompson W, Nielson C, Carvalho P, Charan N, Crowley J (1996) Controlled trial of oral prednisone in outpatients with acute COPD exacerbation. Am J Respir Crit Care Med 154:407–412
45. Davies L, Angus R, Calverley P (1999) Oral corticosteroids in patients admitted to hospital with exacerbations of chronic obstructive pulmonary disease: a prospective randomised controlled trial. Lancet 354:456–460
46. Niewoehner D, Erbland M, Deupree R, et al (1999) Effect of systemic glucocorticoids on exacerbations of chronic obstructive pulmonary disease. Department of Veterans Affairs Cooperative Study Group. N Engl J Med 340:1941–1947
47. Murata G, Gorby M, Chick T, Halperin A (1990) Intravenous and oral corticosteroids for the prevention of relapse after treatment for decompensated COPD: Effect on patients with a history of multiple relapses. Chest 98:845–849
48. Sayiner A, Aytemur ZA, Cirit M, Unsal I (2001) Systemic glucocorticoids in severe exacerbations of COPD. Chest 119:726–730
49. Decramer M, Gosselink R, Troosters T, Verschueren M, Evers G (1997) Muscle weakness is related to utilization of health care resources in COPD. Eur Respir J 10:417–423
50. Woolhouse C, Hill S, Stockley R (2001) Symptom resolution assessed using a patient directed diary card during treatment of acute exacerbations of chronic bronchitis. Thorax 56:947–953
51. Maltais F, Ostinelli J, Bourbeau J, Tonnel A, Jacquemet N, Haddon J (2002) Comparison of nebulized budesonide and oral prednisolone with placebo in the treatment of acute exacerbations of chronic obstructive pulmonary disease: a randomized controlled trial. Am J Respir Crit Care Med 165:698–703
52. Elmes P, Fletcher C, Dutton A (1957) Prophylactic use of oxytetracycline for exacerbations of chronic bronchitis. Br Med J 2:1272–1275
53. Berry D, Fry J, Hindley C, et al (1960) Exacerbations of chronic bronchitis treatment with oxytetracycline. Lancet 1:137–139
54. Elmes P, King T, Langlands J, et al (1965) Value of ampicillin in the hospital treatment of exacerbations of chronic bronchitis. Br Med J 5467:904–908
55. Peterson E, Esmann V, Honcke P, Munkner C (1967) A controlled study of the effect of treatment on chronic bronchitis: an evaluation using pulmonary function tests. Acta Med Scand 182:293–305

56. Pines A, Raafat H, Greenfield J, Linsell W, Solari M (1972) Antibiotic regimens in moderately ill patients with purulent exacerbations of chronic bronchitis. Br J Dis Chest 66:107–115
57. Nicotra MB, Rivera M, Awe RJ (1982) Antibiotic therapy of acute exacerbations of chronic bronchitis. A controlled study using tetracycline. Ann Intern Med 97:18–21
58. Allegre L, Grasi E, Pozzi E (1991) Puolo degli antibiotici nel trattamento delle riacutizza della bronchite cronica. Ital J Chest Dis 45:138–148
59. Nouira S, Marghli S, Belghith M, Besbes L, Elatrous S, Abroug F (2001) Once daily oral ofloxacin in chronic obstructive pulmonary disease exacerbation requiring mechanical ventilation: a randomized placebo-controlled trial. Lancet 358:2020–2035
60. Sachs A, Koeter G, Groenier K, Van Der Waaij D, Schiphuis J, Meyboom-de Jong B (1995) Changes in symptoms, peak expiratory flow, and sputum flora during treatment with antibiotics of exacerbations in patients with chronic obstructive pulmonary disease in general practice. Thorax 50:758–763
61. Sethi S, Paluri R, Grant E, Murphy T (1999) Prediction models for the etiology of acute exacerbations of COPD. Am J Respir Crit Care Med 159:A819 (abst)
62. Stockley R, OBrien C, Pye A, Hill S (2000) Relationship of sputum color to nature and outpatient management of acute exacerbations of COPD. Chest 117:1638–1645
63. Saint S, Bent S, Vittinghoff E, Grady D (1995) Antibiotics in chronic obstructive pulmonary disease exacerbations. A meta-analysis. JAMA 273:957–960
64. Ball P, Harris J, Lowson D, Tillotson G, Wilson R (1995) Acute infective exacerbations of chronic bronchitis. QJM 88:61–68
65. Macfarlane JT, Colville A, Guion A, Macfarlane RM, Rose DH (1993) Prospective study of aetiology and outcome of adult lower-respiratory-tract infections in the community. Lancet 341:511–514
66. Destache CJ, Dewan N, ODonohue WJ, Campbell JC, Angelillo VA (1999) Clinical and economic considerations in the treatment of acute exacerbations of chronic bronchitis. J Antimicrob Chemother 43 (Suppl A):107–113
67. Doern GV, Brueggemann AB, Pierce G, Holley HP Jr, Rauch A (1997) Antibiotic resistance among clinical isolates of Haemophilus influenzae in the United States in 1994 and 1995 and detection of beta-lactamase-positive strains resistant to amoxicillin-clavulanate: results of a national multicenter surveillance study. Antimicrob Agents Chemother 41:292–297
68. Doern G, Pfaller M, Kugler K, Freeman J, Jones R (1998) Prevalence of antimicrobial resistance among respiratory tract isolates of Streptococcus pneumoniae in North America: 1997 results from the SENTRY Antimicrobial Surveillance Program. Clin Infect Dis 27:764–770
69. Sportel JH, Koeter GH, van Altena R, Lowenberg A, Boersma WG (1995) Relation between beta-lactamase producing bacteria and patient characteristics in chronic obstructive pulmonary disease (COPD). Thorax 50:249–253
70. Doern GV, Brueggemann A, Holley HP Jr, Rauch AM (1996) Antimicrobial resistance of Streptococcus pneumoniae recovered from outpatients in the United States during the winter months of 1994 to 1995: results of a 30-center national surveillance study. Antimicrob Agents Chemother 40:1208–1213
71. Doern GV, Pfaller MA, Kugler K, Freeman J, Jones RN (1998) Prevalence of antimicrobial resistance among respiratory tract isolates of Streptococcus pneumoniae in North America: 1997 results from the SENTRY Antimicrobial Surveillance Program. Clin Infect Dis 27:764–770
72. Thornsberry C, Ogilvie P, Kahn J, Mauriz Y (1997) Surveillance of antimicrobial resistance in Streptococcus pneumoniae, Haemophilus influenzae, and Moraxella catarrhalis in the United States in 1996–1997 respiratory season. The Laboratory Investigator Group. Diagn Microbiol Infect Dis 29:249–257
73. Plant PK, Owen JL, Elliott MW (2000) Early use of non-invasive ventilation for acute exacerbations of chronic obstructive pulmonary disease on general respiratory wards: a multicentre randomised controlled trial. Lancet 355:1931–1935

74. Keenan SP, Kernerman PD, Cook DJ, Martin CM, McCormack D, Sibbald WJ (1997) Effect of noninvasive positive pressure ventilation on mortality in patients admitted with acute respiratory failure: a meta-analysis. Crit Care Med 25:1685–1692
75. Mehta S, Hill NS (2001) Noninvasive ventilation. Am J Respir Crit Care Med 163:540–577
76. Anton A, Guell R, Gomex J, et al (2000) Predicting the result of noninvasive ventilation in severe acute exacerbations of patients with chronic airflow limitation. Chest 117:828–833
77. Ambrosino N, Foglio K, Rubini F, Clini E, Nava S, Vitacca M (1995) Non-invasive mechanical ventilation in acute respiratory failure due to chronic obstructive pulmonary disease: correlates for success. Thorax 50:755–757
78. Meduri G, Turner R, Abou-Shala N, Wunderink R, Tolley E (1996) Noninvasive positive pressure ventilation via face mask. First-line intervention in patients with hypercapnic and hypoxemic respiratory failure. Chest 109:179–193
79. Anthonisen N, Connett J, Kiley J, et al (1994) Effects of smoking intervention and the use of an inhaled anticholinergic bronchodilator on the rate of decline of FEV1: The Lung Health Study. JAMA 272:1497–1505
80. Higgins M, Enright P, Kronmal R, Schenker M, Anton-Culver H, Lyles M (1993) Smoking and lung function in elderly men and women. The cardiovascular health study. JAMA 269:2741–2748
81. Postma D, Sluiter H (1989) Prognosis of chronic obstructive pulmonary disease: the Dutch experience. Am Rev Respir Dis 140:S100–S105
82. Wynder E, Kaufman P, Lesser R (1967) A short-term follow-up study on ex-cigarette smokers. With special emphasis on persistent cough and weight gain. Am Rev Respir Dis 96:645–655
83. Rutger S, Postma D, ten Hacken N, et al (2000) Ongoing airway inflammation in patients with COPD who do not currently smoke. Thorax 55:12–18
84. Turato G, Di Stefano A, Maestrelli P, et al (1995) Effect of smoking cessation on airway inflammation in chronic bronchitis. Am J Respir Crit Care Med 152:1262–1267
85. Kanner RE, Anthonisen NR, Connett JE, For the Lung Health STudy Research Group (2001) Lower respiratory illnesses promote FEV1 decline in current smokers but not ex-smokers with mild chronic obstructive pulmonary disease: results from the Lung Health Study. Am J Respir Crit Care Med 164:358–364
86. Fiore M (2000) US public health service clinical practice guidelines: treating tobacco use and dependence. Respir Care 45:1200–1262
87. Jorenby D, Leischow S, Nides M, et al (1999) A controlled trial of sustained-release bupropion, a nicotine patch, or both for smoking cessation. N Engl J Med 340:685–691
88. Buscho R, Saxtan D, Shultz P, Finch E, Mufson M (1978) Infections with viruses and Mycoplasma pneumoniae during exacerbations of chronic bronchitis. J Infect Dis 137:377–383
89. Carilli A, Gohd R, Gordon W (1964) A virologic study of chronic bronchitis. N Engl J Med 270:123–127
90. Lamy M, Ponthier-Simon F, Debacker-Williame E (1973) Respiratory viral infections in hospital patients with chronic bronchitis. Chest 63:336–341
91. Walsh E, Falsey A, Hennessey P (1999) Respiratory syncytial and other virus infections in persons with chronic cardiopulmonary disease. Am J Respir Crit Care Med 160:791–795
92. Smith C, Kanner R, Golden C, Klauber M, Renzetti AJ (1980) Effect of viral infection on pulmonary function in patients with chronic obstructive pulmonary disease. J Infect Dis 141:271–280
93. Nichol K, Margolis K, Wuorenma J, Von Sternberg T (1994) The efficacy and cost effectiveness of vaccination against influenza among elderly persons living in the community. N Engl J Med 331:778–784
94. Nichol K, Baken L, Nelson A (1999) Relation between influenza vaccination and outpatient visits, hospitalizations and mortality among elderly patients with chronic lung disease. Ann Intern Med 130:397–403

95. Fine M, Smith M, Carson C, et al (1994) Efficacy of pneumococcal vaccination in adults. A meta-analysis of randomized controlled trials. Arch Intern Med 154:2666–2677
96. Hutchison B, Oxman A, Shannon H, Lloyd S (1999) Clinical effectivenes of pneumococcal vaccines: Meta-analysis. Can Fam Physician 45:2381–2393
97. Nichol K, Baken L, Wuorenma J, Nelson A (1999) The health and economic benefits associated with pneumococcal vaccination of elderly patients with chronic lung disease. Arch Intern Med 159:2437–2442
98. Butler J, Breiman R, Campbell J, Lipman H, Broome C, Facklam R (1993) Pneomococcal polysaccharide vaccine efficacy: an evaluation of current recommendations. JAMA 270:1826–1831
99. Advisory Committee on Immunization Practices (ACIP) (1997) Prevention of pneumococcal disease. MMWR Recomm Rep 46:1–24
100. Poole P, Black P (2000) Mucolytic agents for chronic bronchitis or chronic obstructive pulmonary disease. Cochrane Database Syst Rev 2:CD001287
101. Stey C, Steurer J, Bachmann S, Medici T, Tramer N (2000) The effects of oral N-acetylcysteine in chronic bronchitis: a quantitative systemic review. Eur Respir J 16:253–262
102. Poole PJ, Black PN (2001) Oral mucolytic drugs for exacerbating of chronic obstructive pulmonary disease: a systemic review. Br Med J 322:1271–1274
103. Grandjean E, Berthet P, Ruffman R, Lenberger P (2000) Cost-effectiveness analysis of oral N-Acetylcysteine as a preventive treatment in chronic bronchitis. Pharmacol Res 42:39–50
104. Abert R, Martin T, Lewis S (1980) Controlled clinical trial of methylprednisolone in patients with chronic bronchitis and acute respiratory insufficiency. Ann Intern Med 92:753–758

Ventilator-associated Pneumonia: What are the Accuracies and the Consequences of Different Diagnostic Methods

A. Torres and S. Ewig

Introduction

Ventilator-associated pneumonia (VAP) is a frequent complication of mechanical ventilation with a crude average incidence of 25%, and it is clearly related to the presence and length of intubation among other important factors. Rates per 1000 ventilator days provides the best comparison and varies from 5 to 35 cases. The mortality of this complication is very high ranging from 30 to 70% and depending on several host and microbial variables. A very important feature related to mortality is the prompt and adequate administration of antibiotics. However, what may seem very simple is in fact rather more complex, as clinicians have to use empirical treatments and microorganisms and their resistances to antibiotics vary frequently from host to host and from unit to unit.

As can be easily understood, obtaining a microbiological diagnosis is the logical first step in the management of VAP. How accurate are the clinical signs and symptoms for suspecting VAP, what is the best method for obtaining respiratory samples, and which are the best types of cultures to perform? These questions and others have been a matter of debate and investigation for the last 15 years. Current thinking about the diagnosis of VAP comes from the following types of study:
1. Observational and comparative studies in a subset of patients with VAP (the most frequent)
2. Observational and comparative studies in patients without VAP (the least frequent)
3. Immediate postmortem studies (in human and animals) to obtain lung samples for culturing and histological examination to be used as a reference test (the most reliable studies).

From the information provided from all these studies four consensus conferences or task-forces (Paris 1990, Memphis 1992, European Task-Force Barcelona 2001, and the Chicago ICU-acquired pneumonia 2002) have been held. In addition, the only evidence-based assessment of diagnostic tests of VAP report was published in Chest in 2000 [1]. The present chapter will be based principally on this publication [1] and will report the opinions of the most recent task-forces or consensus conferences (Barcelona [2] and Chicago [3]). The chapter will be divided into the following sections:

1. Accuracy of tests for diagnosing VAP according to the published evidence,
2. Lessons learnt from post-mortem studies,
3. The information provided from randomized studies
4. Conclusions of the consensus conferences
5. Evidence-based conclusions from the present review.

Accuracy of Tests for Diagnosing VAP According to the Published Evidence

For space limitations we will refer exclusively to the different diagnostic tests to obtain samples for microbiological cultures and to the evidence-based assessment of diagnostic tests for VAP (report of the Clinical Practice Guideline Panel [1]).

Methodology [4]

The evidence based report used strict evidence-based methodology that can be summarized as follows:
- Target condition: VAP.
- Patient population: immunocompetent adults receiving ventilatory support in hospital or long-term care settings. The panel could not address whether testing improves health outcomes.
- Admissible evidence: the evidence considered relevant to the review was prospective or retrospective studies of diagnostic testing in immunocompetent patients with VAP published until 1997. To be admissible, studies had to provide data on sensitivity or specificity or the raw data for calculating them, and a reference standard for how VAP was defined. Pairs of panellists reviewed and summarized the evidence. The MEDLINE database was searched for articles published from 1996 to 1997 by exploding the term pneumonia and the MESH terms "cross infection/artificial ventilation" or the text words "ventilator-associated pneumonia".
- Quality of individual studies: This was judged for internal validity using sample size, selection bias, definition of interventions and outcomes, and confounding variables. Criteria for external validity related to how well the results could be generalized to patients and conditions outside the study settings. Grading systems for judging the quality of evidence typically identified randomized controlled trials as the 'gold standard', followed by controlled observational studies and descriptive epidemiology studies.
- Development of recommendations: This was done according to group discussions based on consideration of the evidence and, when evidence was lacking, on expert opinion.
- The principles for evaluating the diagnostic test performance were the following:
  - *Validity*: Sensitivity, specificity and positive and negative predictive values, numerator and denominator errors (reference standard), blinding and the likelihood ratio. The likelihood ratio is a useful tool for integrating all the information and is defined as the sensitivity divided by 1-specificity. A

likelihood ratio of 9, for example, means that this test would be nine times more likely in patients with pneumonia than in patients without pneumonia.
- Reproducibility which is the ability of a test to yield consistent results when repeated by the same observer

Accuracy of Endotracheal Aspirates [5]

This technique is the simplest non-invasive means of obtaining respiratory secretions from mechanically ventilated patients; it is readily performed at the bedside and requires minimal training of health-care providers. Similar to the sputum, the assessment of the quality of the sample is imperative before processing and has to be done using classical criteria.

From old and more recent literature it is clear that qualitative culturing of endotracheal aspirates are highly nonspecific. Six studies in the literature have investigated the accuracy of quantitative cultures of endotracheal aspirates. The cut-off point established was 100,000-1000000 colony forming units (cfu)/ml. All these studies were prospective and most of them with consecutive enrollment. One study included patients without VAP. Sensitivity ranged from 38 to 82% and the mean sensitivity was 76±9%. Specificity ranged from 72 to 85% and the mean specificity was 75±28 %. The conclusions of the panel [1] were the following:
- The sensitivity and specificity of quantitative tests on cultures of endotracheal aspirate samples vary widely in their ability to diagnose VAP
- Qualitative endotracheal aspirate cultures usually identify organisms found by invasive tests (high sensitivity); however they have a moderate positive predictive value.
- With initial and subsequent episodes of VAP the results of diagnostic tests may vary with the pathogenic bacterial load, the duration of ventilatory support, and antibiotic administration.
- Gram staining and culture of endotracheal aspirate secretions may be useful in diagnosing VAP.

Accuracy of Bronchoalveolar Lavage (BAL) Samples [6]

Quantitative cultures of BAL have been used for many years in the diagnosis of pneumonia. Since the initial description of bronchoscopic BAL in VAP several methodologies have been used that include protected and non-protected systems and different amounts of volumes injected. The cut-off mostly used was 100,000 cfu/ml. The confirmation of the quality of the samples should be done by looking at the percentage of epithelial squamous cells.

Twenty-three studies were reviewed, all of them of prospective nature. Most of them were comparative with other techniques. Several 'gold standards' were used as indicated above. Only two studies looked for squamous epithelial cells as a measure of the quality of the sample. The sensitivity ranged from 42 to 93% and the mean sensitivity was 73±18%. Specificity ranged from 45 to 100% and mean specificity was 82±19 %. The likelihood ratio ranged from 0.9 to 11.6. Twelve studies

looked for the intracellular organism (ICO) detection with a mean sensitivity of 69±20% and a mean specificity of 75±28%. The threshold of ICO detection used ranged from 2 to 5%. The conclusions of the panel [1] were the following:
- The sensitivity of quantitative BAL fluid cultures ranges from 42 to 93 % with a mean of 73%. The clinical implication is that BAL cultures are not diagnostic for pneumonia in almost one fourth of cases.
- The specificity of quantitative BAL fluid cultures ranges from 45 to 100% with a mean of 82%. This means that the diagnosis is incorrect in about 20% of cases.
- Detecting ICO in BAL culture is a quick, specific test and has a high predictive value.
- Only two studies assessed the quality of BAL samples as measured by the presence of squamous epithelial cells.

Accuracy of Protected Specimen Brush Samples (PSB) [7]

The protected specimen brush technique has been used for almost 20 years in diagnosing pneumonia and variations in its methodology have been applied to the diagnosis of VAP. The cut-off point used for quantitative cultures was 103 cfu/ml. The majority of studies reviewed did not control for the quality of samples. Only one study looked at the reproducibility of the technique. This study found that 25% of the time a single PSB determination would have the possibility of being a false-positive or a false-negative. Five out of 18 studies selected used autopsy data from VAP patients as a 'gold standard'. As with other sections most of the studies enrolled the patients prospectively and consecutively. Most of the studies were comparative with other techniques such as endotracheal aspirates and or BAL.

The sensitivity of the technique ranged from 33% to 100% with a mean sensitivity of 66±19 %. The specificity ranged from 50 to 100% with a mean specificity of 90±15%. The likelihood ratio was quite high; the median likelihood ratio was 16. Only one study reported a likelihood ratio <1 and several studies reported ratios > 50 based on a 100% specificity. Interestingly, most of the studies did not describe the risk and complications of the technique. The conclusions of the panel [1] were the following:
- Despite the wide array of studies and the use of high quality diagnostic techniques in several studies to determine the cause of pneumonia, sensitivity ranged from 33 to 100% and specificity ranged from 50 to 100%.
- Overall, PSB appears more specific than sensitive in diagnosing VAP
- In patients with suspected VAP and a positive results of testing a PSB sample, the LR of VAP appears to be much greater than 1.

The Accuracy of Blinded Invasive Diagnostic Procedures in Ventilator-associated Pneumonia [8]

Since fiberoptic bronchoscoy is not exempt of risks and inconveniences other methods of sampling have been developed. The accuracy of these methods is based on the multifocal nature of VAP. Overall three types of blinded methods have been reported: blinded bronchial sampling (BBS), blinded BAL, and blinded use of FSB. The studies used the corresponding cut-off points for each technique. As with studies of other techniques, the patients were enrolled prospectively and consecutively. Again very few studies controlled the quality of the samples and only few studies used the immediate postmorten histology or microbiology for 'gold standard'. There were five studies on BBS, seven studies on mini BAL, and five on blind PBS. The sensitivity varied from 74 to 97% for BBS, from 63 to 100% for miniBAL, and from 58 to 86% for blind PSB. The specificity varied from 74 to 100% for BBS, from 66 to 96% for mini BAL, and from 71 to 100% for blind PSB. The likelihood ratio for the three types of techniques ranged from 2.26 to 18.25.The agreement with fiberoptic techniques (PSB) varied from 73 to 100%. The conclusions of the panel [1] were the following:

- There was a lack of standardization in the type of catheter used, position of the catheter, and in the case of BAL, the volume of fluid instilled.
- The limited number of studies performed to date suggests that the sensitivity and specificity of the blinded techniques is similar to that with fiberoptic bronchoscopy techniques.
- Side effects for blinded techniques appear to be minimal and, at worst, are similar to those for bronchoscopic techniques.

Overall Conclusions from the Panel [1]

Quantitative procedures include non-bronchoscopic techniques and bronchoscopic techniques. Because these tests have similar sensitivities, specificities, predictive values, and likelihood ratios the choice depends on local expertise, experience, availability, and cost factors. The panel recommended formal outcome research with randomized controlled trials to assess various diagnostic and management strategies. This approach would provide the opportunity to evaluate economic outcomes using cost-benefit, cost effectiveness and cost utility analyses.

Lessons Learnt from Postmortem Studies [1, 8]

As we mentioned above, the problem of the 'gold standard' is inherent to most of the studies mentioned above since there is not a clear-cut reference standard. However, those studies that used histology and or microbiology of immediately obtained postmortem lung samples have to be considered as the best. Eleven studies have used this methodology but even among them there was variation about using histology, microbiology or both 'gold standards' to validate diagnostic techniques. These studies should have been done initially when VAP started to be a matter for investigation because from them we learnt several things that could have helped a lot in our understanding on VAP and in the design of 'in vivo' studies.

The main lessons that we learnt from post-mortem studies are the following and have to be used for the interpretation of results obtained 'in vivo':

- VAP is a multifocal process that most frequently involves the lower and posterior segments of the lungs bilaterally.
- VAP is an infectious process in which different phases of severity and evolution coexists. Lung damage is found frequently.
- The quantitative cultures of lung histology cannot discriminate between the absence or the presence of histological pneumonia and they are independent on the evolution period of VAP.
- Prior antibiotic treatment has an important influence on decreasing the lung bacterial burden and consequently influences the positivity or negativity of quantitative cultures according to the thresholds used. In addition, microbes infecting or colonizing lungs from mechanically ventilated patients may be different when comparing different parts of the lungs.
- The multifocal nature of VAP confirms that endotracheal aspirates and BAL samples (in this order) are the best techniques to obtain causative microorganisms of VAP. PSB is a technique that explores a single bronchial segment and has a higher chance for missing causative microorganisms.

Information Provided From Randomized Studies [10-13]

The multicenter French study [10] was a randomized investigation comparing VAP patients managed with invasive quantitative samples (PSB/BAL) versus clinical strategy plus qualitative cultures. The main end points of the study were mortality at day 14 and number of days free of antibiotics. A secondary end point was the frequency of anti-microbial resistance. Studying a total of more than 250 patients, the French investigators found differences in mortality at day 14 (16 vs 26%), in decreasing SOFA score (6 vs 7), and in days free of antibiotics (5 vs 2) in favor of patients managed with invasive strategies compared to these patients that were clinically managed with the help of qualitative endotracheal aspirate cultures. Mortality was not different at day 28. The two main pitfalls of this study were: 1) They used qualitative cultures of endotracheal aspirates, as a comparator, this technique having very poor specificity which consequently leads to overtreatment, to higher numbers of resistant microorganisms, and maybe to a higher mortality. In other words, the results of this study could be easily predicted before the study; 2) In the non-invasive arm there was a significant percentage of inadequate initial treatments that explains and justify part of the differences found in mortality. In practical terms that means that despite patients being randomised, they were not treated equally in terms of empirical antibiotic treatment since there were no differences in microorganisms when comparing both arms. These two important limitations of the study make it useless for the really important question to be answered: do quantitative cultures of invasive techniques influence outcome of patients with VAP?

The Spanish randomized studies [11-13] assessed the influence on outcome when managing patients with quantitative cultures of endotracheal aspirates (except one study that used qualitative cultures [11]) versus those obtained by PSB and/or BAL and they tried to answer the question mentioned above. They could no find differences in mortality, length of stay, or days of mechanical ventilation when comparing patients managed by the invasive or non-invasive strategy. Interestingly, in two studies [12, 13], they used the American Thoracic Society guidelines on hospital-acquired pneumonia [14] to guide initial antibiotic treatments for VAP patients.

A potential pitfall for these studies is that they did not stop antibiotics in the presence of quantitative cultures below the threshold and with clear manifestations of pneumonia. In addition the series were not very large, although all patients together summed more than 200, which is a reasonable figure.

The conclusion of the randomized studies can be summarized as follows:
- Although still unclear, it seems better to manage VAP patients with quantitative cultures of respiratory samples.
- There is no influence on outcome when managing patients with quantitative cultures with or without invasive techniques.

Conclusions of the Consensus Conferences [2, 3]

One recent Task-Force (European Task-Force on VAP [2]) and a Consensus Conference (Consensus Conference on ICU-acquired pneumonia [3]) have given the following conclusions:

a. European Task Force on VAP. What is not controversial:

- Blood cultures are neither sensitive nor specific.
- Qualitative endotracheal aspirates are highly sensitive (75%) but not specific.
- Quantitative cultures of invasive and non-invasive methods are overall sensitive and specific.
- Overall non-bronchoscopic techniques are comparable to bronchoscopic sampling methods.

b. Consensus Conference on ICU-acquired pneumonia.
   Current state of knowledge and unresolved strategies:

- Microbiological samples should be collected before initiation of antimicrobial agents.
- Reliance on endotracheal aspirates leads to both over and under diagnosis of pneumonia.
- Available evidence favors the use of invasive quantitative culture techniques over tracheal aspirates.
- Available data suggests that the accuracy of non-bronchoscopic techniques for obtaining quantitative cultures of lower respiratory tract samples is comparable to that of bronchoscopic techniques.
- The cost-effectiveness of invasive vs non-invasive diagnostic strategies has not been established.

Evidence-based Conclusions from the Present Review

After all the evidence mentioned before we have reached the following conclusions:
a. Quantitative cultures of samples of invasive techniques are not superior to quantitative cultures of endotracheal aspirates. *Category B* (based in two studies).
b. Two randomized studies comparing quantitative cultures of samples from invasive techniques to qualitative cultures of endotracheal aspirates have shown contradictory results. *Category B.*
c. Qualitative cultures of endotracheal aspirates have shown a poor specificity for diagnosing VAP. *Category C*
d. Quantitative cultures of endotracheal aspirates, BAL, PSB, and blind techniques have shown a reasonable sensitivity and specificity. However there is an important variability among studies due to prior antibiotic treatment and the type of 'gold standard' used. The detection of ICO in BAL is a highly specific marker of VAP. None of the methods mentioned above appears to be superior to other in terms of accuracy. *Category C.*

References

1. Grossman R (2000) Evidence-Based assessment of diagnostic tests for ventilator-associated pneumonia: Report of the Clinical Practice Guideline Panel. Chest 117:suppl 2; 177S–218S
2. Torres A, Carlet J (2001) The European Task Force on Ventilator-Associated Pneumonia. Eur Respir J 17:1034–1045
3. Hubmayr RD (2002) Statement of the 4th International Consensus Conference in Critical Care on ICU-Acquired pneumonia. Intensive Care Med 28:1521–1536
4. Woolf SH (2000) Panel methodology: Analytic principles in evaluating the performance characteristics of diagnostic tests for ventilator-associaed pneumonia. Chest 117:182S–185S
5. Cook D, Mandell L (2000) Endotracheal aspiration in the diagnosis of ventilator-associated pneumonia. Chest 17:195S–197S
6. Torres A, El-ebiary M (2000) Bronchoscopic BAL in the diagnosis of ventilator-associated pneumonia. Chest 117:198S–202S
7. Baughman R (2000) Protected specimen brush technique in the diagnosis of ventilator-associated pneumonia. Chest 117:203S–206S
8. Campbell GD (2000) Blinded invasive diagnostic procedures in ventilator-associated pneumonia. Chest 117:207S–211S
9. Rouby JJ (1996) Severe Pulmonary Infections I: Histology and microbiology of ventilator-associated pneumonias. Semin Respir Infect 11:54–61
10. Fagon JY, Chastre J, Wolff M, et al (2000) Invasive and non invasive strategies for management of suspected ventilator-associated pneumonia. A randomized trial. Ann Intern Med 132:621–630
11. Solé-Violan J, Fernández JA, Benítez AB, Cardeñosa JA, Rodríguez de Castro F. Impact of quantitative invasive diagnostic techniques in the mangement and outcome of mechanically ventilated patients with suspected pneumonia. Crit care Med 2000; 28: 2737–2741.
12. Sanchez-Nieto JM, Torres A, Gracía-Cordoba F, et al (1998) Impact of invasive and non invasive quantitative culture sampling on outcome of ventilator-associated pneumonia. Am J Respir Crit Care Med 157:371–376

13. Ruiz M, Torres A, Ewig S, et al (2000) Noninvasive versus invasive microbial investigation in ventilator-associated pneumonia: evaluation of outcome. Am J Respir Crit Care Med 162:119–125
14. American Thoracic Society (1996) Hospital-acquired pneumonia in adults; diagnosis, assessment, initial severity and prevention. A consensus statement. Am J Respir Crit Care Med 153:1711–1725

Are the Most Simple Methods Still Useful in Preventing Respiratory Infections?

E. Girou

Introduction

Pathogens causing nosocomial pneumonia, such as Gram-negative bacilli and *Staphylococcus aureus*, are ubiquitous in healthcare settings, especially in intensive or critical care areas [1]. Transmission of these microorganisms to patients frequently occurs via the hand of healthcare personnel that become contaminated or transiently colonized with the microorganisms [2]. Procedures such as tracheal suctioning and manipulation of ventilator circuit or endotracheal tubes increase the opportunity for cross-contamination. The risk of cross-contamination can be reduced by using aseptic technique and sterile or disinfected equipment when appropriate and eliminating pathogens from the hands of personnel [3].

Hand hygiene is widely recognized as an important but underused measure to prevent nosocomial infections [2]. Even if hand hygiene seems the simplest method of prevention, all studies that have examined handwashing practices for 20 years report great difficulties in obtaining good compliance with this measure. New guidelines that promote the use of handrubbing with a waterless alcohol-based product have been recently published and may increase personnel compliance and decrease incidence of hand-transmitted infections [4].

In this chapter, hand hygiene will refer to the three following techniques: handwashing with a nonmedicated soap or an antiseptic soap, and handrubbing with a waterless alcohol-based product.

Hand Hygiene Reduces Hand Contamination (Category A)

Hand hygiene aims at reducing or eradicating transient flora acquired during patient care activities to avoid cross transmission and thus nosocomial infections. The majority of experimental studies of products for removing transient flora from the hands of healthcare workers involve artificial contamination of the volunteer's skin with a defined inoculum of a test organism before the volunteer uses a plain soap, an antimicrobial soap, or a waterless antiseptic agent. No scientific study has established the extent to which counts of bacteria or other microorganisms on the hands need to be reduced to minimize transmission of pathogens in healthcare facilities; whether bacterial counts on the hands must be reduced by 1 log10 (90% reduction), 2 log10 (99%), 3 log10 (99.9%), or 4 log10 (99.99%) is unknown.

Accepted methods of evaluating hand-hygiene products intended for use by healthcare workers require that test volunteers wash their hands with a plain or antiseptic soap for 30 seconds or 1 minute, despite the observation in the majority of studies that the average duration of handwashing by hospital personnel is <15 seconds [5, 6]. A limited number of investigators have used 15-second handwashing or hygienic hand-wash protocols (Table 1) [4]. Therefore, few data exist regarding the efficacy of hand hygiene under conditions in which they are actually used by healthcare workers. Similarly, certain accepted methods for evaluating waterless antiseptic agents for handrubbing require that 3 ml of alcohol be rubbed into the hands for 30 seconds, followed by a repeat application for the same duration. This type of protocol also does not reflect actual usage patterns among healthcare workers. Furthermore, volunteers used in evaluations of products are usually surrogates for healthcare workers, and their hand flora may not reflect flora found on the hands of personnel working in health-care settings.

As summarized in Table 1, several experimental assays approaching real conditions of use have examined the relative efficacy of hand hygiene techniques to remove micro-organisms from the hands. All showed a poor bactericidal activity of handwashing with nonmedicated soap as compared with hand hygiene with antiseptic agents. To date, only five clinical studies (Table 2) have evaluated the efficacy of hand hygiene procedures in routine practice [7–11].

In a prospective, randomized clinical trial, Zaragoza et al. compared the efficacy of an alcoholic solution with handwashing with nonmedicated soap during regular work in clinical wards and intensive care units (ICUs) of a large public university hospital in Barcelona [11]. Healthcare workers were randomly assigned to handwashing or handrubbing with the alcoholic solution by using a crossover design. The number of colony-forming units (cfu) on agar plates from hand printing in three different samples was counted (before and after hand hygiene procedure, 10 to 30 minutes after hand hygiene procedure). A total of 47 healthcare workers were included. The average reduction in the number of cfu from samples before handwashing to samples after handwashing was 50% for handwashing and 88% for handrubbing. When both methods were compared, the average number of cfu recovered after the procedure showed a statistically significant difference in favor of the alcoholic solution ($p<0.001$). The investigators did not interfere with any healthcare worker during the study. Thus the results reflect the real practice of hand hygiene during care activities.

Pittet et al. performed an uncontrolled observational study to examine the process of bacterial contamination of health care workers' hands during routine patient care in a large teaching hospital. Structured observations of 417 episodes of care were conducted by trained external observers. Each observation period started after a hand hygiene procedure and ended when the healthcare worker proceeded to clean his or her hands or at the end of a coherent episode of care. At the end of each period of observation, an imprint of the five fingertips of the dominant hand was taken and bacterial colony counts were quantified. Regression methods were used to model the intensity of bacterial contamination as a function of method of hand hygiene, duration and type of care, with time of ungloved hands

Table 1. Experimental studies comparing the relative efficacy of nonmedicated soap or medicated soaps versus alcohol-based antiseptics in reducing hand contamination

Authors [Ref]	Year	Skin contamination	Hand sampling method	Time	Relative efficacy
Ayliffe et al. [20]	1978	Artificial contamination	Finger-tip broth culture	30"	UM soap< M soap< ABP
Lilly et al. [21]	1978	Artificial contamination	Finger-tip broth culture	30"	UM soap< M soap< ABP
Ojajärvi et al. [22]	1980	Artificial contamination	Finger-tip broth culture	15"	UM soap< M soap < ABP
Ulrich et al. [23]	1982	Artificial contamination	Glove-juice test	15"	M soap < ABP
Larson et al. [24]	1986	Existing hand flora	Sterile-broth bag technique	15"	UM soap< M soap = ABP
Ayliffe et al. [25]	1988	Artificial contamination	Finger-tip broth culture	30"	UM soap< M soap < ABP
Ehrenkranz et al. [26]	1991	Patient contact	Glove-juice test	15"	UM soap< ABP
Leyden et al.[27]	1991	Existing hand flora	Agar-plate/image analysis	30"	UM soap< M soap < ABP
Namura et al.[28]	1994	Existing hand flora	Agar-plate/image analysis	30"	UM soap< ABP
Paulson et al. [29]	1999	Artificial contamination	Glove-juice test	20"	UM soap< M soap < ABP
Cardoso et al. [30]	1999	Artificial contamination	Finger-tip broth culture	30"	UM soap< M soap< ABP

UM: unmedicated; M: medicated; ABP: alcohol-based product for handrubbing.

during patient care. Respiratory care was a care activity independently associated with higher contamination levels. Simple handwashing with nonmedicated soap before patient care, without hand antisepsis, was also associated with significantly higher colony counts. The major limitation of this study is that observation bias may have accounted for earlier hand hygiene than during routine patient care in the absence of an external observer.

Larson et al. performed a randomized clinical trial to compare skin condition and skin microbiology among 50 ICU personnel using one of two randomly assigned hand hygiene regimens: handwashing with an antiseptic soap or handrubbing with an alcohol-based gel.[8] Each hand hygiene regimen was assigned for four consecutive weeks. Hand cultures (n=193) were obtained four times: at baseline, during the first day of week 1, and as late as possible on the subject's last workday of weeks 2 and 4. For the handwashing group, there were no significant differences between baseline mean log counts and mean log counts from day 1, week 2, or week 4. For the handrubbing group, counts were significantly lower than baseline at day 1 and week 2, but not week 4. The microbial counts on hands of participants using handwashing increased slightly in weeks 2 and 4, whereas the counts decreased slightly at each time interval among those using handrubbing. However, the timing of hand cultures was questionable in this study whose primary endpoint was not to asses hand hygiene efficacy. In a similarly designed randomized clinical trial, Lucet et al. did not find a significant difference in bacterial counts between antiseptic handwashing and handrubbing [9].

In a randomized controlled trial, Girou et al. compared the efficacy of handrubbing with an alcohol based solution versus conventional handwashing with antiseptic soap in reducing hand contamination during routine ICU patient care [7]. During daily nursing sessions of 2 to 3 hours, 23 healthcare workers were randomly assigned to either handrubbing with alcohol based solution or handwashing with antiseptic soap when hand hygiene was indicated before and after patient care. Imprints were taken of fingertips and palm of dominant hand before and after hand hygiene procedure. Bacterial counts were quantified blindly and 114 patient care activities were evaluated. With handrubbing, the median percentage reduction in bacterial contamination was significantly higher than with handwashing (83 v 58%, P=0.012), with a median difference in the percentage reduction of 26% (95% confidence interval, 8 to 44%). The major limitation of this trial is that the sampling method may have underestimated the degree of contamination in both groups.

With regard to this body of data coming from experimental and clinical studies, handrubbing with an alcohol-based product appears to be the best method to achieve hand disinfection.

Hand Hygiene Reduces Nosocomial Infections (Category C)

Studies evaluating the impact of hand hygiene on nosocomial infection rates examine generally all sites of infection together. Therefore, no study has measured specifically the impact of hand hygiene on respiratory infections. In some studies, the results are detailed according to the site of infection, but, usually, they are not powered enough to evidence significant differences by site of infection. Most of

Table 2. Clinical studies assessing the effectiveness of hand hygiene to reduce hand contamination

Authors [Ref]	Year	Study design	Study location	Main results
Zaragoza et al. [11]	1999	Randomized controlled study	Hospital	Handrubbing > Handwashing with NMS
Pittet et al. [10]	1999	Uncontrolled observational study	Hospital	Handrubbing > Handwashing with NMS
Larson et al. [8]	2000	Randomized controlled study	Adult ICU	Handrubbing = Handwashing with AS
Lucet et al. [9]	2002	Randomized controlled study	Adult ICU	Handrubbing = Handwashing with AS
Girou et al. [7]	2002	Randomized controlled study	Adult ICU	Handrubbing > Handwashing with AS

NMS: nonmedicated soap; AS: antiseptic soap.

the studies presented below took advantage of the discovery of poor hand hygiene practices to evaluate interventions aimed at increasing hand hygiene compliance, and monitored nosocomial infection rates in parallel. Such studies are very difficult to perform because the duration of follow-up has to be long to see both increase in compliance and decrease in infections.

An intervention trial using historical controls demonstrated in 1847 that the mortality rate among mothers who delivered in the First Obstetrics Clinic at the General Hospital of Vienna was substantially lower when hospital staff cleaned their hands with an antiseptic agent than when they washed their hands with nonmedicated soap and water [12]. Semmelweis observed that the mortality rate of puerperal fever was substantially higher in the First Clinic (16%) where doctors and medical students provided care to women in labor as compared with the Second Clinic (7%) where midwives assisted at all deliveries. He postulated that the high rate of puerperal fever was caused by "cadaverous particles" transmitted from the autopsy rooms to the obstetrics ward via the hands of students and doctors despite washing them with unmedicated soap and water. In May 1847, Semmelweis insisted that students and doctors scrub their hands in a chlorinated lime solution before every physical examination. The maternal mortality rate in the First Clinic subsequently dropped dramatically to 3% in the 7 remaining months of 1847 and remained low for years. This intervention by Semmelweis represents the first evidence that cleansing heavily contaminated hands with an antiseptic agent between patient contacts can reduce nosocomial transmission of contagious diseases more effectively than handwashing with nonmedicated soap and water.

In 1977, Casewell et al. found that 70% of the staff of an adult ICU had their hands contaminated with *Klebsiella* [13]. These strains could be related to serotypes infecting or colonizing patients in the ward on the same day. They identified ward procedures that resulted in contamination of nurses' hands with 10^2 to 10^3 *Klebsiella* per hand with a survival on hands for up to 150 minutes. Handwashing with an antiseptic agent reliably gave 98–100% reduction in hand counts, and the introduction of routine handwashing by staff before moving from one patient to the next was associated with a significant and sustained reduction in the number of patients colonized or infected with *Klebsiella*. However, the investigators did not quantitate the level of handwashing compliance among personnel.

In a sequential comparative trial of three handwashing agents in a surgical ICU (i.e., nonmedicated soap and two antiseptic soaps, each regimen used exclusively for approximately six weeks), the incidence of nosocomial infection was 50% lower during the use of the antiseptic handwashing products than during the use of nonmedicated soap (p<0.001) [14].

With a sequential intervention study in an ICU, Conly et al. demonstrated that poor handwashing practices were associated with a high nosocomial infection rate, whereas good handwashing practices were associated with a low nosocomial infection rate [15]. An educational program designed to improve handwashing procedures significantly reduced endemic nosocomial infection rates. Before the educational program, the nosocomial infection rate (number of infections per 100 patient discharges) was greater than 30% with handwashing compliances of 14 and 28% before and after patient contact, respectively. After the institution of the first educational program, the infection rate decreased dramatically to 12% meanwhile handwashing compliance rates reached 73 and 81% before and after contact. The infection rates were maintained low during the three subsequent years. The fourth year, nosocomial infection rates increased to 33% with poor handwashing practices (26 and 23% before and after contact, respectively). A second educational program was implemented, and nosocomial rates dropped again to 9% with average handwashing compliance of 60%.

Handwashing and infection rates were studied in two ICUs of a community teaching hospital [16]. Handwashing rates were monitored secretly throughout the study. After six months of observation, educational interventions were started to increase handwashing. Handwashing increased gradually, but overall compliance rates before (22%) and after (30%) interventions were not significantly different (p=0.07) whereas infection rates per 100 admissions remained stable (22% and 23%).

For eight months, Doebbeling et al. conducted a prospective multiple-crossover trial involving 1894 adult patients in three ICUs [17]. In a given month, the ICU used a hand-washing system involving either chlorhexidine or alcohol, with the optional use of a nonmedicated soap; in alternate months the other system was used. Rates of nosocomial infection and handwashing compliance were monitored prospectively. When chlorhexidine was used, there were 152 nosocomial infections, as compared with 202 when the combination of alcohol and soap was used (adjusted incidence-density ratio [IDR], 0.73; 95% confidence interval, 0.59 to 0.90). The largest reduction with chlorhexidine was in gastrointestinal infections. However, because only a minimal amount of the alcohol rinse was used during periods when the combination regimen also was in use and because compliance with handwashing instructions was higher when chlorhexidine was available (48 versus 30%, p=0.002), determining which factor (i.e., the hand-hygiene regimen or differences in adherence) accounted for the lower infection rates was difficult.

Webster et al. evaluated hand wash products in terms of user acceptability and effectiveness against methicillin-resistant S. aureus (MRSA) as part of a long-term strategy to eliminate endemic MRSA from the neonatal ICU at an Australian hospital [18]. Following the introduction of a new hand wash disinfectant, new cases of MRSA colonization were monitored for 12 months. In addition, the use of antibiotics, the incidence of multi-resistant Gram-negative cultures, and neonatal infections were noted. No changes were made to any procedures or protocols during the trial. All babies colonized with MRSA were discharged from the nursery within 7 months of the introduction of triclosan and in the subsequent 9 months no new MRSA isolates were reported. Compared with the previous 12 months, fewer antibiotics were prescribed and fewer nosocomial infections recorded (p<0.05).

Zafar et al. described nosocomial infections due to MRSA of 22 male infants in a neonatal nursery during a 7-month period and the infection control procedures that effectively brought this outbreak under control and eliminated recurrence for more than 3 years [19]. After a single index case of bullous impetigo caused by MRSA in a neonate discharged from the nursery 2 weeks previously, an additional 18 cases of MRSA skin infections were clustered in a 7-week period. Aggressive infection control measures were instituted, including changes in umbilical cord care, circumcision procedures, diapers, handwashing, gloves, gowns, linens, disinfection, placement in cohorts of neonates and staff, surveillance, and monitoring. These measures were not effective in slowing the outbreak. The single additional measure of changing handwashing and bathing soap to a preparation containing an antiseptic (0.3% triclosan) was associated with the immediate termination of the acute phase of the MRSA outbreak.

Impact of Hand Hygiene Promotion on Nosocomial Infection Rates (Table 3)

Pittet et al. attempted to promote hand hygiene by implementing a hospital-wide program, with special emphasis on bedside, alcohol-based hand disinfection and measuring nosocomial infections in parallel. The overall compliance with hand hygiene during routine patient care in a teaching hospital in Geneva, was monitored before and during implementation of a hand-hygiene promoting campaign. Seven hospital-wide prevalence surveys were done twice yearly from December, 1994, to December, 1997. Secondary outcome measures were nosocomial infection rates, attack rates of MRSA, and consumption of handrub disinfectant. Compliance with hand hygiene improved progressively from 48% in 1994, to 66% in 1997 (p<0.001). During the same period, overall nosocomial infection decreased (prevalence of 17% in 1994 to 10% in 1998; p=0.04), MRSA transmission rates decreased (2.16 to 0.93 episodes per 10,000 patient-days; p<0.001), and the consumption of alcohol-based handrub solution increased from 3.5 to 15.4 l per 1000 patient-days between 1993 and 1998 (p<0.001).

Table 3. Clinical studies evaluating the impact of hand hygiene promotion on nosocomial infection rates

Authors [Ref]	Year	Study design	Study location	Impact on Hand Hygiene Compliance	Impact on nosocomial infections rates
Casewell et al. [13]	1977	Non-randomized controlled study	Adult ICU	NM	↘ Klebsiella infections
Maki et al. [14]	1989	Non-randomized controlled study	Adult ICU	NM	↘ infections
Conly et al. [15]	1989	Non-randomized controlled study	Adult ICU	↗	↘ infections
Simmons et al. [16]	1990	Non-randomized controlled study	Adult ICU	No effect	No effect
Doebbeling et al. [17]	1992	Non-randomized controlled study	Adult ICU	↗	↘ infections
Webster et al. [18]	1994	Non-randomized controlled study	Neonatal ICU	NM	↘ MRSA cross transmission
Zafar et al. [19]	1995	Non-randomized controlled study	Neonatal ICU	NM	↘ MRSA cross transmission
Pittet et al. [31]	2000	Non-randomized controlled study	Hospital	↗	↘ infections
					↘ MRSA cross transmission
Larson et al. [32]	2000	Non-randomized controlled study	Hospital	↗	↘ VRE cross transmission

NM: not monitored; MRSA: methicillin-resistant *Staphylococcus aureus*; VRE: vancomycin-resistant enterococci. ↗ significant increase; ↘ significant decrease.

Larson et al. conducted a quasi-experimental intervention trial to assess the impact of an intervention to change behavior on frequency of staff handwashing (as measured by counting devices inserted into soap dispensers on four ICUs) and nosocomial infections associated with MRSA and vancomycin-resistant enterococci (VRE). All staff in one of two hospitals received an intervention with multiple components designed to change behavior; the second hospital served as a comparison. Over a period of 8 months, 860,000 soap dispensings were recorded, with significant improvements in the study hospital after 6 months of follow-up. Rates of MRSA were not significantly different between the two hospitals, but rates of VRE were significantly reduced in the intervention hospital during implementation.

Conclusion

In conclusion, there is a good level of evidence showing that hand hygiene with antiseptic products is effective to reduce hand contamination significantly during patient care activities. Surely, the best technique is handrubbing with an alcohol-based solution. This measure should decrease the risk of cross transmission of microorganisms and thus decrease the risk of acquiring an infection, especially in ICU patients. However, the level of evidence demonstrating a link between an increased compliance to hand hygiene and low rates of nosocomial infections is low according to the classification used in this chapter. Good evidence for effect of a procedure should be obtained from placebo-controlled, double-blind, crossover studies. For obvious reasons, no such studies on the effect of hand hygiene in ICUs ever have been or will be performed. Hand hygiene has been general practice in medical care since the days of Semmelweis. No ethics committee would accept a study where some intensive care patients intentionally received care from staff with dirty hands!

The hand hygiene research agenda should certainly include valid epidemiological research generating more definitive evidence for the impact of improved compliance with hand hygiene on infection rates [2]. But also, and maybe as a priority, the key determinants of hand-hygiene behavior must be assessed and the evidence-based indications for hand cleansing must be promoted among the different populations of healthcare workers, (considering that it might be unrealistic to expect healthcare workers to clean their hands after every patient contact), the necessary percentage increase in hand-hygiene compliance resulting in a predictable risk reduction in infection rates.

References

1. Alberti C, Brun-Buisson C, Burchardi H, et al (2002) Epidemiology of sepsis and infection in ICU patients from an international multicentre cohort study. Intensive Care Med 28:108-121.
2. Pittet D, Boyce JM (2001) Hand hygiene and patient care: pursuing the Semmelweis legacy. Lancet Infect Dis 0:9–20
3. Hubmayr RD (2002) Statement of the 4th international consensus conference in critical care on ICU-acquired pneumonia – Chicago, Illinois, May 2002. Intensive Care Med 28:1521–1536
4. Boyce JM, Pittet D, Healthcare Infection Control Practices Advisory Committee (2002) Guidelines for hand hygiene in health-care settings: Recommendations of the Healthcare Infection Control Practices Advisory Committee and the HICPAC/SHEA/APIC/IDSA Hand Hygiene Task Force. MMWR Recomm Rep 51:1–45
5. Gould D (1994) Nurses' hand decontamination practice: results of a local study. J Hosp Infect 28:15–30
6. Lund S, Jackson J, Leggett J, Hales L, Dworkin R, Gilbert D (1994) Reality of glove use and handwashing in a community hospital. Am J Infect Control 22:352–357
7. Girou E, Loyeau S, Legrand P, Oppein F, Brun-Buisson C (2002) Efficacy of handrubbing with an alcohol-based solution versus standard handwashing with an antiseptic soap. A randomised clinical trial. Br Med J 325:362–366
8. Larson EL, Aiello AE, Bastyr J, et al (2001) Assessment of two hand hygiene regimens for intensive care unit personnel. Crit Care Med 29:944–951

9. Lucet JC, Rigaud MP, Mentre F, et al (2002) Hand contamination before and after different hand hygiene techniques: a randomized clinical trial. J Hosp Infect 50:276–280
10. Pittet D, Dharan S, Touveneau S, Sauvan V, Perneger TV (1999) Bacterial contamination of the hands of hospital staff during routine patient care. Arch Intern Med 159:821–826
11. Zaragoza M, Sallés M, Gomez J, Bayas JM, Trilla A (1999) Handwashing with soap or alcoholic solutions? A randomized clinical trial of its effectiveness. Am J Infect Control 27:258–261
12. Semmelweis I (1983) Etiology, concept, prophylaxis of childbed fever. 1st ed. The University of Wiscosin Press, Madison
13. Casewell M, Phillips A (1977) Hands as route of transmission for Klebsiella species. Br Med J 2:1315–1317
14. Maki DG (1989) The use of antiseptics for handwashing by medical personnel. J Chemother 1:3–11
15. Conly JM, Hill S, Ross J, Lertzman J, Louie TJ (1989) Handwashing practices in an intensive care unit: The effects of an educational program and its relationship to infection rates. Am J Infect Control 17:330–339
16. Simmons B, Bryant J, Neiman K, Spencer L, Arheart K (1990) The role of handwashing in prevention of endemic intensive care unit infections. Infect Control Hosp Epidemiol 11:589–594
17. Doebbeling BN, Stanley GL, Sheetz CT, et al (1992) Comparative efficacy of alternative hand-washing agents in reducing nosocomial infections in intensive care units. N Engl J Med 327:88–93
18. Webster J, Faoagali JL, Cartwright D (1994) Elimination of methicillin-resistant *Staphylococcus aureus* from a neonatal intensive care unit after hand washing with triclosan. J Paediatr Child Health 30:59–64
19. Zafar AB, Butler RC, Reese DJ, Gaydos LA, Mennonna PA (1995) Use of 0.3% triclosan (Bacti-Stat) to eradicate an outbreak of methicillin-resistant *Staphylococcus aureus* in a neonatal nursery. Am J Infect Control 23:200–208
20. Ayliffe GAJ, Babb JR, Quoraishi AH (1978) A test for "hygienic" hand disinfection. J Clin Pathol 31:923–928
21. Lilly HA, Lowbury EJL (1978) Transient skin flora: their removal by cleansing or disinfection in relation to their mode of deposition. J Clin Path 31:919–922
22. Ojajärvi J (1980) Effectiveness of hand washing and disinfection methods in removing transient bacteria after patient nursing. J Hyg (London) 85:193–203
23. Ulrich JA (1982) Clinical study comparing hibistat (0.5% chlorhexidine gluconate in 70% isopropyl alcohol) and betadine surgical scrub (7.5% povidone-iodine) for efficacy against experimental contamination of human skin. Curr Ther Res 31:27–30
24. Larson EL, Eke PI, Laughton BE (1986) Efficacy of alcohol-based hand rinses under frequent-use conditions. Antimicrob Agents Chemother 30:542–544
25. Ayliffe GAJ, Babb JR, Davies JG, Lilly HA (1988) Hand disinfection: a comparison of various agents in laboratory and ward studies. J Hosp Infect 11:226–243
26. Ehrenkranz NJ, Alfonso BC (1991) Failure of bland soap handwash to prevent hand transfer of patient bacteria to urethral catheters. Infect Control Hosp Epidemiol 12:654–662
27. Leyden JJ, McGinley KJ, Kaminer MS, et al (1991) Computerized image analysis of full-hand touch plates: a method for quantification of surface bacteria on hands and the effect of antimicrobial agents. J Hosp Infect 18:13–22
28. Namura S, Nishijima S, Asada Y (1994) An evaluation of the residual activity of antiseptic handrub lotions: an "in use" setting study. J Dermatol 21:481–485
29. Paulson DS, Fendler EJ, Dolan MJ, Williams RA (1999) A close look at alcohol gel as antimicrobial sanitizing agent. Am J Infect Control 27:332–338
30. Cardoso CL, Pereira HH, Zequim JC, Guilhermetti M (1999) Effectiveness of hand-cleansing agents for removing acinetobacter baumannii strain from contaminated hands. Am J Infect Control 27:327–331

31. Pittet D, Hugonnet S, Harbath S, et al (2000) Effectiveness of a hospital-wide programme to improve compliance with hand hygiene. Lancet 356:1307–1312
32. Larson EL, Early E, Cloonan P, Sugrue S, Patrides M (2000) An organizational climate intervention associated with increased handwashing and decreased nosocomial infections. Behavior Med 26:14–22

Tracheostomy in Patients with Respiratory Failure Receiving Mechanical Ventilation: How, when, and for whom?

C. Apezteguia, F. Ríos, and D. Pezzola

Introduction

Tracheostomy is probably the most frequent surgical procedure performed on intensive care unit (ICU) patients. About 10–11% of critically ill patients receiving mechanical ventilation require tracheostomy [1]. Most of these patients need ventilatory support for a long time, or have been identified by the physician as potentially requiring mechanical ventilation for an extended period. Consequently, patients with neuromuscular diseases are tracheostomized more often and earlier than patients with chronic obstructive pulmonary disease (COPD); and the latter more frequently and earlier than acute respiratory failure patients [4]. The principal argument to tracheostomize these patients is to avoid lesions produced by prolonged translaryngeal intubation. Other valuable benefits include easy tube reinsertion, better secretion removal, and improved patient comfort and mobility. The disadvantages of tracheostomy comprise perioperative complications related to the procedure and the patient's condition, long-term airway injury, and the cost of the intervention. There are also doubts concerning the actual effects on patient outcome, the best technique to carry out the procedure, the most appropriate timing, and the facilitating role on the weaning process, amongst other uncertainties.

The Consensus conference on artificial airways in patients receiving mechanical ventilation [5] recognized the existing gaps in knowledge on the subject and established the need for further research. However, some general recommendations were given, e.g., to favor indication of tracheostomy for anticipated need of artificial airway for longer than 21 days and to discourage it for anticipated need of up to 10 days, with daily assessment for intermediate situations. In his position paper, Heffner stresses that the ideal clinical study comparing the risks and benefits of tracheostomy vs. prolonged translaryngeal intubation has not yet been done, and emphasizes the need to individualize medical decisions according to the patient's clinical condition.

We will now review the available literature on several issues related to this intervention. Some of the answers needed to improve the management of patients receiving mechanical ventilation should be drawn from the following questions:

1. What is the outcome of patients who receive a tracheostomy?
2. When should tracheostomy be performed?

3. On whom should tracheostomy be performed?
4. Can tracheostomy facilitate weaning?
5. How should tracheostomy be performed? Are non-surgical techniques safer than standard surgical tracheostomy?

The objective of this chapter is to systematically review the literature that addresses these questions.

Focus of the Review

We reviewed the published information (meta-analyses, randomized trials, controlled non-randomized studies and the clinically most applicable observational trials) that may help in the management of mechanically ventilated critically ill patients. We excluded editorials, letters, narrative reviews, case reports, and articles restricted to cost analysis.

We were interested in heterogeneous ICU patients receiving mechanical ventilation. Our target population included adult patients who underwent a tracheostomy while receiving mechanical ventilation. The clinical settings relevant to our review included ICUs and intermediate-care units. We excluded studies of home ventilation, those using chronic ventilation settings, tracheostomy aimed at facilitating terminal or palliative care, and studies of highly specific populations (e.g., patients with chronic spinal cord diseases, spinal cord injury, head and neck tumors, craniofacial abnormalities, maxillofacial lesions or sleep breathing disorders).

For the technical aspects of the procedure, we included studies that addressed the controversy between surgical and non-surgical techniques, but we did not include differences between non-surgical techniques and cricothyroidotomy.

Search for Relevant Studies

We conducted a comprehensive search for the relevant studies, with no language restriction, in MEDLINE, Cumulative Index to Nursing and Allied Health Literature (CINAHL), the Cochrane Controlled Trials Registry and the Cochrane Data Base of Systematic Reviews, and the system Literatura Latino Americana y del Caribe de Información en Ciencias de la Salud (LILACS) from 1972 to August 2002. We examined the reference lists of all included articles for other potentially relevant citations and personal files. In MEDLINE, the terms "tracheotomy" and "tracheostomy" were used as Medical Subject Headings (MeSH terms) and were also searched in titles and abstracts. Citations were limited to human studies. We did not explicitly search for unpublished literature, but known unpublished studies were considered. We retrieved all articles that any of the three reviewers considered potentially eligible according to the titles and abstracts. The same reviewers examined the full text and jointly made the final decisions regarding eligibility, based on the inclusion and exclusion criteria described above.

Data Assessment

We examined all eligible articles regarding methodological features (summary in Table 1). When a meta-analysis or systematic review was selected, the trials evaluated in it were not reanalyzed. When more than one meta-analysis or systematic review examined the same or almost the same articles, only the study with the best methodological characteristics was selected. In cases of duplicate studies, only one of the trials was included. Types of studies selected for each of the subjects analyzed were different, according to the characteristics of the articles found in the search. We used critical appraisal questions for most studies taken from the *Users' Guides to the Medical Literature* series published in the *Journal of the American Medical Association*. The level of evidence was classified as categories A, B, C or D, according to the system developed by the NHLBI.

Results

Out of the 4136 articles originally searched, 791 articles meeting the requirements of the selection criteria were retrieved from the database. Only 115 proved potentially eligible on the basis of reviewing the title and abstract. We eventually included a total of 15 studies after a comprehensive review of the full article. Regarding `general outcome', two observational controlled studies were included. For `timing (early vs. late)', we included a systematic review, a randomized controlled trial and an observational controlled trial. Only four studies on physiological outcome before/after tracheostomy, indirectly informing on facilitation of `weaning', were included due to lack of available literature about clinical outcomes. Two meta-analysis and four randomized controlled trial about `techniques' addressing complications were included. Methodological characteristics and the number of patients studied in each article are summarized in Table 1.

General Outcome

In the case-control study by Esteban et al [1] of 373 tracheostomized patients (10.7%) as an integral part of the trial data of 5081 patients receiving mechanical ventilation [6], the tracheostomized patients were matched with 373 patients without tracheostomy of similar characteristics. Tracheostomy was performed at a median of 12 (7, 17) days after the beginning of mechanical ventilation; in 53.2% of the cases during the weaning period, and in 29.7% after extubation followed or not by reintubation. Risk factors associated with tracheostomy were duration of mechanical ventilation, reintubation, coma, and neuromuscular disease. The tracheostomy group had longer ICU length of stay (26.9 vs. 11.7 days) and hospital length of stay (43.8 vs. 22.1 days). Tracheostomy resulted in reduction of ICU mortality (24.4 vs. 37.3%; relative risk 0.65) but did not modify hospital mortality (38.6 vs. 41.6%; relative risk 0.93).

To identify clinical predictors and outcomes for tracheostomy in ICU patients, Kollef et al [2] studied 51/521 mechanically ventilated patients that had a tra-

Table 1. Summary of methodological characteristics of studies and number of patients included

Item	Esteban 2001 [1]	Kollef 1999 [2]	Maziak 1998 [7]	Sugerman 1997 [8]	Brook 2000 [9]	Diehl 1999 [10]	Davis 1999 [11]	Lin 1 1999 [12]	Mohr 2001 [13]	Dulguerov 1999 [14]	Freeman 2000 [15]	Heikkinen 2000 [16]	Freeman 2001 [17]	Massick 2001 [18]	Melloni 2002 [19]
Study	Case-control	Prospective observational	Systematic review	RCT multi-center	Prospective observational	Before/after trial	Before/after trial	Before/after trial	Before/after trial	Meta-analysis	Meta-analysis	RCT	RCT	RCT	RCT
Clear-cut objectives	Yes	Yes	Yes	Yes	Yes	Yes	Yes	Yes	Yes	Yes	Yes	Yes	Yes	Yes	Yes
Randomization	No	No	Partial	Yes, but reassignment	No	No	No	No	No	No	Partial	Yes	Yes	Yes	Yes
Inclusion/exclusion criteria	Yes	Yes	Yes	Yes	Yes	Yes	Yes	Yes	Yes	Yes	Yes	Yes	Yes	Yes	Yes
Similarities between groups	Yes	Partial	–	Partial	Partial	Yes	Yes	Yes	Yes	–	–	Yes	Yes	Yes	Partial
Dropouts accounted for	Not stated	Not stated	–	Yes	Not tated	Not stated	Not stated	Not stated	Yes	–	–	Not stated	Not stated	Not stated	Not stated
Follow-up	Hospital discharge	1 m after hospital	–	3–5 m, incomplete	Hospital discharge	–	–	–	–	–	–	18 m, incomplete	Hospital discharge	Hospital discharge	6 m
Statistical analysis	Yes	Yes	Yes	Yes	Yes	Yes	Yes	Yes	Yes	Yes	Yes	Yes	Yes	Yes	Yes
Explicit search methods	–	–	Yes	–	–	–	–	–	–	Yes	Yes	–	–	–	–

Table 1. Continued

Item	Esteban 2001 [1]	Kollef 1999 [2]	Maziak 1998 [7]	Sugerman 1997 [8]	Brook 2000 [9]	Diehl 1999 [10]	Davis 1999 [11]	Lin 1 1999 [12]	Mohr 2001 [13]	Dulguerov 1999 [14]	Freeman 2000 [15]	Heikkinen 2000 [16]	Freeman 2001 [17]	Massick 2001 [18]	Melloni 2002 [19]
Study	Case-control	Prospective observational	Systematic review	RCT multicenter	Prospective observational	Before/after trial	Before/after trial	Before/after trial	Before/after trial	Meta-analysis	Meta-analysis	RCT	RCT	RCT	RCT
Inclusion criteria	–	–	Yes	–	–	–	–	–	–	Yes/Not stated	Yes	–	–	–	–
Assessing validity of studies															
Similarities between studies	–	–	No	–	–	–	–	–	–	No	Partial	–	–	–	–
Conclusions according to the evidence reviewed	–	–	Yes	–	–	–	–	–	–	Yes	Yes	–	–	–	–
n pts group T/ group NT*	373/373	51/470	–	74/74	–	8/8	20/20	20/20	45/45	3512/1817 (+4185)	121/115	–	–	–	–
N pts group ET/ group LT**	–	–	163/ 156+?	53/21	53/37	–	–	–	–	–	–	26/30	40/40 ?	–	–
n pts group SgT/ group NSgT***	–	–	–	–	–	–	–	–	–	–	–	–	–	50/50 (+64)	25/25

* Pts. group T/group NT: Group of patients with tracheostomy/Group of patients without tracheostomy
** Pts. group ET/group LT : Group of patients with early tracheostomy/Group of patients with late tracheostomy
*** Pts. group SgT/group NSgT: Group of patients with surgical tracheostomy/Group of patients with non-surgical tracheostomy
RCT: randomized controlled trial

cheostomy (9.8%) placed 9.7 ± 6.4 days after the onset of mechanical ventilation. Risk factors for receiving a tracheostomy were nosocomial pneumonia, aerosol therapy, witnessed aspiration, and reintubation. Tracheostomy patients had longer ICU (18.8 vs. 5.7 days) and hospital (30.9 vs. 12.8 days) lengths of stay. Hospital mortality was less than the mortality of the non-tracheostomy group (13.7 vs. 26.4%, relative risk 0.52), but this effect was restricted to medical patients. The authors concluded that, despite having longer lengths of stay in the ICU and hospital, patients with respiratory failure who received a tracheostomy had favorable outcomes compared with patients who did not.

Timing: Early versus late tracheostomy

Maziak et al. [7] published a systematic review with clearly defined inclusion/exclusion criteria, where they carefully analyzed five articles subjected to a rigorous validity assessment. The reviewers showed the heterogeneity between studies (three were quasi-RCTs and two retrospective studies, different populations, unequal definitions of early and late) and concluded there is insufficient evidence to support that the timing of tracheotomy alters the duration of mechanical ventilation or the extent of airway injury in critically ill patients.

Sugerman et al. [8] in their multicenter randomized controlled trial, after a drop out of 20% of the patients, entered 112 to early randomization (3–5 days) and 14 to late randomization (10–14 days); an additional 22 patients from the early entry groups were re-randomized late. The comparisons were made between the tracheostomy and non-tracheostomy groups in each scenario: early (three diagnostic groups) and late. Although there was a higher APACHE III score in the early tracheostomy group than in the early non-tracheostomy group, the authors did not find significant differences in ICU length of stay, frequency of pneumonia, or death in any of the groups after either early or late tracheostomy compared with continued endotracheal intubation. However, computing ICU length of stay among tracheostomized patients, it is shorter in the early surgery group than in the late tracheostomy group (20 ± 2 vs. 38 ± 5 days, $p = 0.0008$). A total of 124 patients underwent laryngoscopy at endotracheal extubation or at tracheostomy removal; there were no significant differences between the groups. The endoscopic follow-up at 3 to 5 months was scarce.

In the prospective observational study by Brook [9], 53 patients were examined who had tracheostomy done by day 10 of mechnaical ventilation (5.9 ± 7.2 days) and 37 had late tracheostomy (16.7 ± 2.9 days). Male sex (OR 3.84 [2.32–6.34]) and higher PaO_2/FiO_2 ratios (OR 1.01 [1.00–1.01]) were associated with early tracheostomy. In the early tracheostomy group, a briefer period of mechanical ventilation (28.3 ± 28.2 days vs. 34.4 ± 17.8 days; $p = .005$) was observed and a reduction in ICU length of stay (15.6 ± 9.3 days vs. 29.3 ± 15.4 days; $p < .001$) but not in hospital length of stay. Timing of tracheostomy was not associated with occurrence of nosocomial pneumonia or hospital mortality.

Facilitation of Weaning

Diehl et al. [10] compared work of breathing (WOB), intrinsic positive end-expiratory pressure (PEEPi), and breathing pattern in eight ventilator-dependent patients before and after tracheotomy. These measurements were performed at different levels of pressure support and tracheostomy decreased resistive and elastic work of braething in most of them, more definitely when the ventilator support was diminished. Significant reductions in occlusion pressure and PEEPi were also observed, without significant changes in breathing pattern. The percentage of ineffective efforts decreased after tracheostomy in the three patients who had these events prior to surgery. An *in-vitro* part of the study showed that the cannula lowered the resistive work induced by the endotracheal tube. The conclusion of the authors was that tracheostomy can substantially reduce the mechanical workload of ventilator dependent patients.

In 20 patients judged ready for extubation in whom extubation failed on two occasions, Davis et al. [11] measured respiratory mechanics, breathing pattern, and work of breathing during spontaneous breathing, before and after tracheostomy. After tracheostomy, work of breathing per minute (8.9 ± 2.9 vs. 6.6 ± 1.4 J/min; $p = 0.04$), and intrinsic PEEP (2.9 ± 1.7 vs. 1.6 ± 1.0 cm H_2O; $p = 0.02$) were reduced. All patients were successfully weaned from the ventilator within 24 hours of tracheostomy. The authors believe that the rigid nature of the tracheostomy tube represents reduced imposed work of breathing compared with the longer, thermolabile endotracheal tube. These findings, however, do not fully explain the ability of patients to be liberated from mechanical ventilation after tracheostomy.

Lin et al. [12] studied 20 chronic lung disease patients under prolonged mechanical ventilation for pulmonary mechanics and breathing pattern under mechanical ventilation, pre and post tracheostomy; four of them with preceding weaning failure. They could find no significant differences except for reduction in the peak inspiratory pressure. In a *post hoc* analysis of pre-tracheostomy values in the group that could be weaned and the patients that were not weaned in two weeks, the weaned patients had lower PEEPi and larger static compliance.

Pulmonary mechanics, breathing pattern, arterial blood gases, and capnography with determination of dead space ventilation (Vd/V_T) were measured in 45 surgical patients under mechanical ventilation by Mohr et al. [13]. There was no difference noted in any of the measures pre and post-tracheostomy. On subgroup analysis, those patients that were weaned from mechanical ventilation with 72 hours of tracheostomy were compared with those patients weaned from mechanical ventilation 5 days or more after tracheostomy and, again, no difference was found.

Surgical versus Non-surgical Technique

The meta-analysis by Dulguerov et al. [14] is a very extensive one that includes prospective and observational studies. It comprises 17 older articles (1960–1984) on surgical tracheostomy alongside 21 more recent (1985–1996) trials on surgical tracheostomy, and 27 others on non-surgical tracheostomy (percutaneous). Comparison of recent surgical and non-surgical tracheostomy trials, showed that perioperative complications are more frequent with the percutaneous technique (10% vs. 3%), whereas postoperative complications occur more often with surgical tracheostomy (10% vs. 7%). Among major complications, perioperative death (0.44% vs. 0.03%) and serious cardiorespiratory events (0.33% vs. 0.06%) were higher with non-surgical tracheostomy. There was heterogeneity in the articles for the analysis of complications. According to authors, percutaneous tracheostomy is associated with a higher prevalence of perioperative complications, whereas postoperative complication rates are higher with surgical tracheostomy.

Freeman et al. [15] published a meta-analysis pooling the data of five trials directly comparing surgical with percutaneous dilational tracheostomy (PDT). Operative time was shorter for PDT and there was no difference regarding overall operative complication rates. However, PDT was associated with less perioperative bleeding (OR 0.14 [0.02–0.39]) and lower overall postoperative complication (bleeding, stomal infection) rate (OR 0.14 [0.07–0.29]). No difference was identified in overall procedure-related complications or death. The authors concluded that this meta-analysis suggests potential advantages of PDT relative to surgical tracheostomy in the appropriately selected critically ill patient.

In a randomized controlled study [16], 30 patients underwent PDT and 27 patients had surgical tracheostomy. All tracheostomies were performed at the patient's bedside in the ICU. The mean time to perform PDT was shorter. Five patients in the PDT group and one in the surgical tracheostomy group had moderate bleeding during the procedure or perioperatively. Although they performed surgical tracheostomy at the bedside in the ICU to avoid the risks associated with moving critically ill patients to the operating room, authors found PDT to be a simple and safe procedure.

Freeman et al. [17] in their randomized controlled trial addressing cost-effectiveness, compared PDT (performed in the ICU) and surgical tracheostomy (in the operating room). PDT was performed more quickly and there were no differences in ICU length of stay or hospital length of stay. There were two patients of the surgical tracheostomy group with serious hemorrhages, and a trend was registered to greater mortality in the group (PDT 22.5%; surgical 45%, p = 0.06). According to the authors, PDT may become the procedure of choice for electively establishing tracheostomy in the appropriately selected patient who requires long-term mechanical ventilation.

Massick et al. [18] analyzed the complication incidence of two methods of bedside tracheostomy: Surgical tracheostomy (50 patients) or endoscopically guided PDT (50 patients); 64 other patients did not meet the selection criteria for non-surgical tracheostomy and received surgical trachestomy in the operating room. This operating room group had significantly increased perioperative complication rates compared with those patients who met selection criteria for bedside tracheostomy (20 vs. 5%, p ≤ 0.01). No statistically significant difference was found in the perioperative complication incidence between the two methods of bedside tracheostomy. However, PDT resulted in a significant increase in postoperative complications (16 vs. 2%, $p < .05$) including one case of death related to tube displacement. Conclusion of the authors: this investigation prospectively confirms the safety of bedside tracheostomy placement in properly selected patients, even when open surgical tracheostomy represents the standard of care in bedside tracheostomy placement by providing a more secure airway.

Melloni et al. [19] compared the effects of surgical tracheostomy versus PDT under fiberoptic control on complication rates, in particular late tracheal complications up to 6 months. PDT was performed faster than surgical tracheostomy. There were no differences in intraoperative complications. Early postoperative complications, particularly stomal infections, occurred more frequently in the surgical group (36 vs. 4%). Although the difference was not statistically significant, in the surgical group there were no late tracheal complications, whereas in the PDT group, two late tracheal complications (one segmental malacia and one stenosis at the level of the stoma) were observed. According to the authors, this study confirms that PDT is a simpler and quicker procedure than surgical tracheostomy and that it has a lower rate of early postoperative complications.

Discussion

The frequency of tracheostomy in the management of the patient receiving mechanical ventilation contrasts with the lack of clear evidence as regards how to perform it. Recommendations of the Consensus Conference of 1989 [5], founded basically by expert opinion, are not often respected in current practice and the physician frequently makes decisions based on his/her own preferences. In this chapter, we have reviwed some of the most conflicting issues related to this procedure.

The characteristics of the studies selected were dissimilar, depending on the search results for each subject analyzed. In the field of techniques, there is an acceptable representation of meta-analysis and randomized controlled trials with definite clinical outcomes. Conversely, for weaning there is a lack of relevant clinical trials and only articles with physiologic end-points could be selected. General outcome and timing field were represented by an intermediate situation.

General Outcome

Retrieving the available information on prognosis and current practice is relevant in the gathering of the knowledge needed to base decision-making on the management of critically ill patients. Such information also provides a basis for assessing best practice standards.

Two well designed controlled observational trials were selected: the study by Esteban et al. [1], a case-control study using high-grade data from a prospective, multicenter, international, very large trial, and the article by Kollef et al. [2], that showed results of the practice performed in a single hospital. Both studies show important aspects on these issues.

Ten to eleven percent of ICU patients receiving mechanical ventilation have a tracheostomy. Its frequency increases with duration of mechanical ventilation, need for reintubation, presence of coma or neuromuscular disease, nosocomial pneumonia, aerosol therapy, and aspiration. The timing observed was 12 (or 10) days from the beginning of mechanical ventilation, occurring earlier in neurologic and trauma patients, and with a high frequency during weaning or after extubation. Tracheostomy patients had longer ICU and hospital stays in both studies. Mortality in the ICU was lower than in the non-tracheostomy group, but hospital mortality was the same [1]. Kollef et al. found that hospital mortality was lower in the tracheostomy group than in the non-tracheostomy group. This finding can be explained because some patients died before reaching a long enough duration of mechanical ventilation to be elegible for tracheostomy. Consequently, the number of deaths in the non-tracheostomy group is enlarged, thus creating a systematic bias for higher survival of the tracheostomy group compared with the non-tracheostomy group.

In summary, in current practice, tracheostomy is provided to 11% of ICU patients under mechanical ventilation, increasing with length of mechanical ventilation, need for reintubation, presence of coma or neuromuscular disease. The procedure is performed at a median of 12 days of mechanical ventilation, and earlier in neurologic or trauma patients. Most cases of tracheostomy are done during weaning or after extubation. The population of tracheostomized patients has longer stays in the ICU and in the hospital than non-tracheostomy patients; their hospital mortality is 39%, similar to the non-tracheostomy patients, but ICU mortality is lower *(Level of evidence category C)*.

Timing: Early Versus Late Tracheostomy

This is a controversial subject, probably due to the lack of convincing evidence about the relative importance of airway lesions induced by translaryngeal intubation and tracheostomy, the uneven duration of mechanical ventilation in different illnesses, its influence on weaning, chances to be discharged from the ICU, etc.

The systematic review of Maziak et al. [7] is constrained by studies that show various weaknesses; their analysis concludes that there is insufficient evidence to support that timing alters the duration of mechanical ventilation or extent of airway injury. The multicente randmoized controlled trial by Sugerman et al. [8] has a confounding randomization and a design that diversifies the groups, making it difficult to compare between early (53 patients) and late (21 patients) tracheostomy groups. Despite the authors' assertion that "there were no significant differences in ICU length of stay, frequency of pneumonia, or death", the early tracheostomy group had a briefer ICU length of stay. There were no differences in laryngeal lesions during hospitalization but the late tracheostomy group follow up was scarce. The observational study by Brook et al. [9] found a briefer period of mechanical ventilation and ICU length of stay, but not in hospital length of stay, for the early tracheostomy group. Timing was not associated with nosocomial pneumonia or hospital mortality. Regrettably, these new trials from Maziak's review do not add sufficient evidence about timing to answer the question.

In summary, there is not convincing evidence to support that early tracheostomy modifies mortality, airway injury, occurrence of nosocomial pneumonia, or hospital length of stay. Probably, it can diminish the duration of mechanical ventilation and ICU loength of stay *(Level of evidence category C)*.

Facilitation of Weaning

Among the studies on late tracheostomy to facilitate weaning, which show apparently divergent results, that by Diehl et al. [10] stands out as a most methodologically careful article studying a small number of patients under different levels of ventilatory support. It shows that tracheostomy decreased resistive and elastic work of breathing and PEEPi, more markedly with less ventilatory support. Moreover, the shorter length of the tracheal tube and the reduction of the inner diameter of the endotracheal tube owing to inspissated secretions may explain the decrease of resistive load after tracheostomy. The study by Davis et al. [11] displays an attractive design: a population composed of patients deemed ready for extubation in whom extubation had previously failed, with measurements done during spontaneous breathing, pre and post tracheostomy. As with Diehl´s study, work of breathing and PEEPi appeared reduced after tracheostomy.

Concerning the other two studies with negative results, that by Lin et al. [12] measured patients receiving mechanical ventilation that was set independently of the study and was not 'normalized' and that by Mohr et al. [13] practiced determinations in patients ventilated with intermittent mandatory ventilation (IMV) at a 10/min rate combined with pressure support. Probably these conditions of 'heavy' ventilatory support veiled the change in work of breathing induced by tracheostomy.

In summary, although no studies demonstrate enhanced weaning from mechanical ventilation in patients with tracheostomy compared with translaryngeal intubation, the former procedure is associated with diminished work of breathing and PEEPi in patients requiring low levels of ventilatory support (*Level of evidence category C)*

Surgical Versus Non-surgical Technique

This is a specially evolving field because the recently incorporated non-surgical techniques, including percutaneous dilatational (Ciaglia or Griggs techniques and their variants) and translaryngeal tracheostomy, are in direct competition with the long-established procedure of standard surgical tracheostomy. Furthermore, some non-surgical techniques have already been discontinued and others are undergoing changes and adaptations in search of the optimal procedure. The learning curve of any new surgical procedure correlates with a decreasing trend in the occurrence of related complications. Another aspect to be considered is the fact that the technique selected usually determines the location where the procedure is performed: Surgical tracheostomy in the operating room and non-surgical tracheostomy in the ICU. Other items are the need of a 'normal neck anatomy' to use percutaneous techniques and the procedure restrictions due to patient condition (abnormalities of coagulation, high level of PEEP, etc).

We limited our analysis to articles that compare surgical with non-surgical tracheostomy: two meta-analysis and four randomized controlled trials. Both meta-analyses can be the subject of technical criticism, principally the vast review by Dulguerov et al. [14] that pooled, in a single statistical analysis, very many heterogeneous studies over an extended time span. In their data, the incidence of perioperative complications varied with differing non-surgical techniques, including some that are no longer on the market because of their high complication rates. Freeman's review [15], a reasonably well conducted meta-analysis, compares surgical tracheostomy with only one non-surgical technique, PDT, in prospective trials. Not all the studies were randomized and the complication rates of the different studies are quite variable, so the level of heterogeneity among the studies could be a question. The findings of Dulguerov and colleagues suggest disadvantages of non-surgical with respect to surgical tracheostomy concerning perioperative complications, including death. On the contrary, the findings of Freeman et al. show less perioperative bleeding with PDT. In both meta-analyses, overall postoperative complication are lower with non-surgical techniques.

Regarding the moderate sample sized randomized controlled trials, all four trials compare surgical tracheostomy (bedside or in the operating room) with PDT (in the ICU) and all but Heikkinen's study [17] performed PDT under endoscopic vision. The trials do not show differences in perioperative complications except for Freeman's study [16], which does register two serious hemorrhages in the surgical group. Regrading postoperative complications, although Melloni et al. [19] finds that stomal infections occurred more frequently in the surgical group, Massick et al. [18] noted that PDT resulted in a significant increase incidence with one case of death. There is agreement among the authors that PDT is a simple, quick and quite safe procedure. Freeman et al. [16] consider that it may become the procedure of choice in the appropriately selected patient, while Massick et al. [18] state that open surgical tracheostomy represents the standard of care in bedside tracheostomy placement by providing a more secure airway. Finally Massick et al. and Freeman et al. emphasize the need to define criteria for patients eligible for bedside non-surgical tracheostomy (neck anatomy, coagulation, PEEP, ease to intubate).

According to the evidence examined, we can establish some statements for surgical tracheostomy versus PDT. It can be stated that there are no differences in perioperative complications apart from more frequent hemorrhages in surgical tracheostomy. Regarding early postoperative complications, their frequency is less in PDT than in surgical tracheostomy although scarce reports show fatal complications in the non-surgical group. Even though PDT can be a simple, quick and quite safe procedure when used in the appropriately selected patient, particularly under endoscopic control, surgical tracheostomy is the procedure of choice to provide a more secure airway in the critically ill patient who does not comply with the selecting criteria for non-surgical tracheostomy *(Level of evidence category B)*.

Future Research

The present review of the published data discloses the need to conduct new, adequately powered prospective studies focusing on the clinical outcomes in several areas. Studies could be improved by using more rigorous patient inclusion and exclusion criteria, better accountability for dropouts, conventional randomization methods, multicenter designs that allow for sufficient sample sizes to determine the interaction of underlying conditions, and multivariate analysis tech-

niques [20]. Large randomized controlled trials are necessary and these trials must be comprehensive of different interrelated topics.
1. There is no conclusive evidence about the relative contribution of translaryngeal intubation and tracheostomy to various early and late complications: cardiorespiratory events, airway lesions, occurrence of nosocomial pneumonia, and accidental extubation or decannulation.
2. The question of timing remains unresolved. It is necessary to compare outcomes for patients randomized to mechanical ventilation via long term translaryngeal intubation versus early conversion to tracheostomy, beginning with groups of patients that are prone to benefit from an `early approach' (neuromuscular disease, neurologic diseases with sensorial impairment, cranioencefalic trauma).
3. The current practice of doing a tracheostomy to facilitate weaning from a ventilator in a patient that is difficult to wean has not been clinically demonstrated. A protocol to verify this presumption is clearly needed.
4. A large trial is required to compare different techniques: standard surgical tracheostomy, Ciaglia procedure, Griggs technique, and translaryngeal tracheostomy, with definite inclusion/exclusion criteria.

Acknowledgment. The authors thanks Jorge Roca for his assistance with the preparation of the manuscript.

References

1. Esteban A, Frutos F, Anzueto A, et al (2001) Impact of tracheostomy on outcome of mechanical ventilation. Am J Respir Crit Care Med 163:A129 (abst)
2. Kollef MH, Ahrens TS, Shannon W (1999) Clinical predictors and outcomes for patients requiring tracheostomy in the intensive care unit. Crit Care Med 27:1714–1720
3. Fischler L, Erhart S, Kleger GR, Frutiger A (2000) Prevalence of tracheostomy in ICU patients. A nation-wide survey in Switzerland. Intensive Care Med 26:1428–1433
4. Esteban A, Anzueto A, Alía I, et al (2000) How is mechanical ventilation employed in the intensive care unit? An international utilization review. Am J Respir Crit Care Med 161:14501458
5. Plummer AL, Gracey DR (1989) Consensus conference on artificial airways in patients receiving mechanical ventilation. Chest 96:178184
6. Esteban A, Anzueto A, Frutos F, et al (2002) Characteristics and outcomes in adult patients receiving mechanical ventilation. A 28-day international study. JAMA 287:345–355
7. Maziak DE, Meade MO, Todd TR (1998) The timing of tracheotomy: a systematic review. Chest 114:605–609
8. Sugerman HJ, Wolfe L, Pasquale MD, et al (1997) Multicenter, randomized, prospective trial of early tracheostomy. J Trauma 43:741–747
9. Brook AD, Sherman G, Malen J, Kollef MH (2000) Early versus late tracheostomy in patients who require prolonged mechanical ventilation. Am J Crit Care 9:352–359
10. Diehl JL, Atrous SE, Touchard D, Lemaire F, Brochard L (1999) Changes in the work of breathing induced by tracheotomy in ventilator-dependent patients. Am J Respir Crit Care Med 159:383388
11. Davis, K Jr, Campbell, RS, Johannigman JA, Valente JF, Branson RD (1999) Changes in Respiratory Mechanics After Tracheostomy. Arch Surg 134:59-62

12. Lin MC, Huang CC, Yang CT, Tsai YH, Tsao TC (1999) Pulmonary mechanics in patients with prolonged mechanical ventilation requiring tracheostomy. Anaesth Intensive Care 27:581–585
13. Mohr AM, Rutherford EJ, Cairns BA, Boysen PG (2001) The role of dead space ventilation in predicting outcome of successful weaning from mechanical ventilation. J Trauma;51:843848
14. Dulguerov P, Gysin C, Perneger TV, Chevrolet JC (1999) Percutaneous or surgical tracheostomy: a meta-analysis. Crit Care Med 27:1617–1625
15. Freeman BD, Isabella K, Lin N, Buchman TG (2000) A meta-analysis of prospective trials comparing percutaneous and surgical tracheostomy in critically ill patients. Chest 118:1412–1418
16. Freeman BD, Isabella K, Cobb JP, et al (2001) A prospective, randomized study comparing percutaneous with surgical tracheostomy in critically ill patients. Crit Care Med 29:926–930
17. Heikkinen M, Aarnio P, Hannukainen J (2000) Percutaneous dilational tracheostomy or conventional surgical tracheostomy? Crit Care Med 28:1399–1402
18. Massick DD, Yao S, Powell DM, et al (2001) Bedside tracheostomy in the intensive care unit: a prospective randomized trial comparing open surgical tracheostomy with endoscopically guided percutaneous dilational tracheotomy. Laryngoscope 111:494–500
19. Melloni G, Muttini S, Gallioli G, et al (2002) Surgical tracheostomy versus percutaneous dilatational tracheostomy. A prospective-randomized study with long-term follow-up. J Cardiovasc Surg (Torino) 43:113–121
20. Heffner JE (2001) The role of tracheotomy in weaning. Chest 120:477S–481S

The Use of Sedation and Neuromuscular Blockade: The Effect on Clinical Outcome

B. De Jonghe, B. Plaud, and H. Outin

Introduction

Sedatives and neuromuscular blockers are widely used in intensive care units (ICUs), especially in patients receiving mechanical ventilation [1]. The main objective of sedation is to increase patient comfort and tolerance to the ICU environment, particularly the ventilator [2]. Tracheal intubation, ventilator mode and setting, and tracheal suction largely contribute to discomfort, pain, ventilator dyssynchrony, and anxiety in mechanically-ventilated patients. The most important deleterious effects of sedatives are a delayed recovery of consciousness after the acute phase of illness, and prolongation of mechanical ventilation and ICU stay. These may also be further increased by concomitant administration of neuromuscular blockers, which are used to treat organ dysfunction in severely ill patients [3], but may also lead to prolonged neuromuscular blockade, and the development of axonal or myopathic changes [4].

The aim of this chapter was to systematically review the effects of different sedation and neuromuscular blockade drugs and strategies on patient comfort, recovery of clinical neuromuscular function and duration of mechanical ventilation and ICU stay.

Methods

To identify studies, we searched MEDLINE from January 1966 to July 2002, using the following text words and key words: "sedation" or "neuromuscular blockers" or "comfort" or "tolerance" or "anxiety" or "agitation" or "weaning" or "neuromuscular" or "artificial ventilation" or "ICU"or "intensive care" or "critically ill". In the Cochrane Library, we searched both the Clinical Trials Registry for randomized trials and the Cochrane database of Systematic Reviews. We identified and retrieved relevant articles from the reference lists of all primary articles and review articles, and those in our personal files.

The following selection criteria were applied:
1. **Population:** adult ICU patients with invasive or non-invasive mechanical ventilation

2. **Endpoints:** comparative effects of intravenous (IV) sedatives or competitive neuromuscular blockers on the following outcomes: patient comfort, pain or anxiety and consciousness (for sedatives only); duration of weaning, mechanical ventilation, stay in ICU; clinical recovery of neuromuscular function (recovery based on train-of-four (TOF) stimulation was not selected). For studies comparing 2 sedatives, only comparisons between midazolam and propofol were selected.
3. **Design:** Eligible studies were published as full-text articles with the following design: prospective controlled interventional studies and meta-analysis of prospective randomized controlled trials. Studies included in meta-analyses were not analyzed separately.

Data on the population, the sedatives or neuromuscular blockers used, measured outcomes, and type of study design were abstracted. Studies were classified into one of the following categories: comparison of two sedatives or neuromuscular blocking drugs and comparison of two sedation or neuromuscular blockade strategies

Results

Of the 12 studies identified, four (including one meta-analysis [5]) compared sedative drugs [5–8], four compared sedation strategies [9–12], three compared neuromuscular blockade strategies [13–15], and one compared a combined sedation and neuromuscular blockade strategy [16]. No study comparing two neuromuscular blockers drugs was identified according to the above criteria. Study characteristics and results are reported in Table 1.

Studies Comparing the Effect of Two Different Sedatives or Neuromuscular Blockers on Selected Outcomes

One meta-analysis aggregated the results of 17 prospective randomized controlled trials comparing midazolam with propofol [5]. The time spent at the target sedation level was 2.9 h longer (significant difference) with propofol compared to midazolam. In the 12 studies of short-term sedation included in this meta-analysis, the weaning time (defined as the interval between discontinuation of sedation and successful extubation) was 2.2 h shorter (significant difference) with propofol compared to midazolam.

In patients receiving mid- or long-term sedation, the effect of midazolam vs propofol on weaning time was evaluated in five comparisons reported in three studies [6–8] representing 197 patients. A significant reduction in mean weaning time with propofol (up to 49 h) was found in the five comparisons. Time to ICU discharge in the propofol group was significantly reduced in two comparisons [6], but significantly prolonged in two others [8].

Studies Comparing the Impact of Two Sedation or Neuromuscular Blockade Strategies on the Selected Outcome.

Of the five studies which compared a conventional sedation strategy with a protocol-based sedation strategy, two were prospective randomized controlled trials [9, 10]. In the first study, the sedation protocol consisted of frequent reassessment of patients sedation requirements and active tapering of the infusion rate [9]. The second study evaluated the daily interruption of sedatives and reassessment of patient needs [10]. Protocol-based sedation was associated with a significant reduction in duration of mechanical ventilation, ICU stay, and hospital stay in both studies [9, 10]. Of the three prospective studies which compared the periods before and after implementation of the sedation protocol [11, 12, 16], two (one of which assessed both an analgesia and a TOF-based neuromuscular blockade algorithm along with the sedation algorithm [16]) showed a reduction in duration of mechanical ventilation [12, 16], whereas in the third, a trend to longer weaning time and time to discharge from ICU was observed in algorithm-directed sedation groups [11]. In the latter study, the effect of the sedation algorithm on the quality of sedation was comprehensively evaluated. Implementation of the sedation protocol resulted in a significant reduction in Ramsay 1 events (patients agitated or anxious or both) and increase in Ramsay 4 events (patients showing a brisk response after a light glabellar tap) [11].

In the single identified study comparing intermittent "as needed" bolus doses vs continuous infusion of neuromuscular blockers, fewer patients had persistent severe muscle weakness after pancuronium discontinuation in the "as needed" IV bolus group compared to the continuous infusion group (with TOF target 1 or 2) [13]. However, the total number of patients who were assessed for weakness was not provided. A prospective randomized controlled trial comparing TOF-based vs "as needed" administration of continuous IV neuromuscular blockers showed that continuous IV administration of vecuronium with TOF monitoring was associated with a significant 2.8 hour reduction in time to spontaneous ventilation [14]. In a prospective, controlled, non-randomized trial, the TOF-protocol group showed a shorter duration of mechanical ventilation after paralysis than the "as needed" group (3.7 vs 8.5 days), but the difference was not statistically significant [15].

Discussion

Midazolam and propofol have been compared in numerous prospective, randomized, controlled trials [17]. A large meta-analysis showed that time spent on adequate sedation might be longer (up to 3 hours) with propofol than with midazolam [5]. However, the relevance of this short clinical difference is questionable. In studies of short-term sedation, a shorter time to extubation with propofol was also identified. Again the clinical relevance of this difference is uncertain. Furthermore, most of these short-term sedation studies were conducted in post-cardiac surgery patients, which precludes generalization to general ICU populations.

Table 1. Impact of sedation drugs and strategies on the selected outcomes.

Category	Study	Design	Population	Endpoints	Analysis Midazolam	Analysis Propofol	P value	Comments
Propofol compared to midazolam	Walder 2001 [5]	Meta-analysis of PRCTs	17 PRCTs (short-, mid- or long-term sedation)	Duration of adequate sedation, h	Weighted mean difference = 2.9 h (0.2 – 5.6) in favor of propofol		0.04	Large majority of short-term sedation studies in post-operative patients (cardiac surgery)
			Short term sedation (<36h): 12 PRCTs N=663	Weaning time, h	Weighted mean difference = 2.2 h (0.8 – 3.7) in favor of propofol		significant	Significantly more arterial hypotension and hypertriglyceridemia episodes in propofol patients.
	Carrasco 1993 [6]	Interventional PCRT	N=28 General ICU Sedation 24h – 1 wk No CNS disorders	Time to extubation, h Time to ICU discharge	13.5 ± 4.0 21.0 ± 5.8	0.4 ± 0.1 1.4 ± 0.5	<0.05 <0.05	Ramsay sedation scale, target 2-3-4-5 and GCS modified by Cook & Palma, target 8-13
.			N=20 General ICU Sedation >1 wk No CNS disorders	Time to extubation, h Time to ICU discharge, h	36.6 ± 6.8 54.7 ± 12.3	0.8 ± 0.3 1.8 ± 0.7	<0.05 <0.05	Sedation algorithm: ± Weaning protocol: ±
	Barrientos-Vega 1997 [7]	Interventional PCRT	N=108 General ICU No CNS disorders Mean sedation time: 140.7 h	Time to 1st T-piece trial, h Time to extubation, h	48.9 ± 47.2 97.9 ± 54.6	4.0 ± 3.9 34.8 ± 29.4	0.0001 <0.0001	Ramsay sedation scale, target 4-5 Sedation algorithm: ± Weaning protocol: ±
	Hall 2001 [8]	Interventional PRCT Multicentric	N=99 General ICU No CNS disorders	Time to extubation, h Time to ICU discharge, h %time at target Ramsay	24.7 (14.5-35.0) 63.7 (44.3-80.0) 44.0% (35.0-52.9)	6.7 (4.2-9.1) 94.0 (44.0-143.9) 60.2 % (52.6-67.9)	NA NA <005	Individualized target on Ramsay sedation scale
.			Sedation <24h, N=58	Time to extubation, h Time to ICU discharge, h	9.1 (5.5-12.7) 33.7 (24.3-43.1)	6.3 (3.4-9.2) 43.4 (30.9-55.9)	0.17 0.22	Sedation algorith: no
			Sedation 24-72 h N=15	Time to extubation, h Time to ICU discharge, h	31.0 (6.3-55.7) 76.7 (29.7-123.7)	9.9 (1.3-18-5) 156.5 (0-335.8)	0.014 0.008	
.			Sedation 72 h N=26	Time to extubation, h Time to ICU discharge, h	52.7 (25.6-79.8) 121.7 (63.1-180.3)	5.3 (1.4-9.2) 154.7 (0-316.6)	0 0.004	Weaning protocol: no

Table 1. Continued.

Category	Study	Design	Population	Endpoints	Analysis Conventional Sedation	Analysis Algorithm-directed sedation	P value	Comments
Sedation algorithm compared to no algorithm	Brook 1999 [9]	Interventional PCRT	N=321 Medical ICU	MV duration, h tracheostomy ICU LOS, d Hospital LOS, d	124.0± 153.6 21/159 (13.2%) 7.5 ± 6.5 19.9 ± 24.2	89.1 ± 133;6 10/162 (6.2%) 5.7 ± 5.9 14.0 ± 17.3	0.003 0.038 0.013 <0.001	DZP or MDZ bolus, LZP infusion Ramsay sedation scale, target 3 Weaning protocol: yes Quality of sedation measured: no
	Kress 2000 [10]	Interventional PCRT	N=128 Medical ICU	MV duration, d ICU LOS, d Hospital LOS, d	7.3 (3.4-16.1) 9.9 (4.7-17.9) 16.9 (8.5-26.6)	4.9 (2.5-8.6) 6.4 (3.9-12.0) 13. (7.3-20.0)	0.004 0.02 0.19	MDZ or propofol Ramsay sedation scale, target 3-4 Weaning protocol: no Quality of sedation measured: no
	McLaren 2000 [11]	Prospective, Interventional Controlled (before-after)	N=158 Medical-surgical-neurological ICU	Time to extubation, h Time to ICU discharge, h Ramsay 1 events Ramsay 4 events	39.1 ± 54.7 111.9 ± 121.1 22.4 % 17.2 %	61.6 ± 97.4 114.6 ± 115 11.0 % 29.6 %	0.13 NS $P<0.001$ $P<0.01$	LZP, MDZ and PPF Modified Ramsay sedation scale, individualized target Weaning protocol: no
	Brattebo 2002 [12]	Prospective, Interventional Controlled (before-after)	N=285 Surgical ICU	MV duration, d ICU LOS, d	7.4 (7.5) 9.3 (8.7)	5.3 (4.5) 8.3 (7.5)	Significant NS	Algorithm not provided MAAS sedation scale Weaning protocol: no Quality of sedation measured: no
	Mascia 2000 [16]	Prospective, Interventional Controlled (before-after)	N= 156 General ICU	MV duration, h ICU LOS, d Hospital LOS, d Alive and full function at discharge	317 19.1 34.3 22.2%	167 9.9 23.3 65.5%	NA NA NA <0.0001	3 specific algorithms (Sedation, analgesia & NMB use) Ramsay sedation scale, target: 2 PPF, MDZ and LZP Weaning protocol: no Quality of sedation measured: no

PRCT: prospective, randomized trial; CNS: central nervous system; MV: mechenaical ventilation; ICU intensive care unit; LOS: length offf stay; NMB: neuromuscular blockade; PPF: propofol; DZP: diazepam; MDZ: midazolam; LZP: lorazepam

Table 2. Impact of neuromuscular blockade strategies on the selected outcomes.

Category	Study	Design	Population	Endpoints	Analysis		P value	Comments
					Continuous IV strategy	Repeated IV bolus "as clinically needed" strategy		
Continuous vs bolus strategy for NMB administration	De Lemos 1999 [13]	Prospective interventional Controlled Not randomized	N=30 General ICU Pancuronium (mean duration: 6 days) no renal failure and no CNS disorder	Persistent severe muscle weakness (total number of patients assessed not reported)	n=5	n=1	NA	Numerous methodological problems acknowledged by the authors continuous IV strategy: TOF target 1 or 2 on 4
					As clinically needed	TOF		
TOF-based vs "as clinically needed" strategy for continuous infusion of NMB	Rudis 1997 [14]	Interventional PRCT 2 centers	N=77 Medical ICUs Vecuronium (mean duration: 50 h)	Time to spontaneous ventilation, median, h	4.8 (3.0-9.0)	2.0 (1.6-5.0)	0.047	TOF target in TOF group: 1 on 4
				Weakness at recovery of TOF 4/4* assessed in 42 of the 65 patients who survived the paralytic episode	17/20 85.0%	13/22 59.1%	NS	Risk for delayed return to spontaneous ventilation in the "as clinically needed" group in creased in patients with renal failure or administration of aminoglycosides or corticosteroids
				Prolonged weakness (until death or hospital discharge)	3	1	NS	
	Strange 1997 [15]	Prospective interventional Controlled Not randomized	N=36 Medical ICU, Atracurium (mean duration: 125 h)	Onset of first muscular movement, min	45 ± 12	50 ± 10	0.74	High TOF target (3 on 4) in TOF group;
				Time to extubation, d	8.5 ± 3.1	3.7 ± 1.3	0.13	"As clinically needed" strategy included daily return to limb movement

LOS: length of stay; ICU: intensive care unit; MV: mechanical ventilation; NS: non significant; NA: not available; PRCT: prospective randomized controlled trial; MDZ: midazolam; TOF: train-of-four

In patients receiving long-term sedation with propofol, time to extubation was markedly shorter compared to those receiving midazolam [6-8]. However, compared to the important number of ICU patients receiving sedation for 48 hrs each year, very few patients have been studied to date. Furthermore, because of the particular physical characteristics of propofol, none of these studies was double-blinded. This may have introduced a bias in the decision to extubate or discharge a patient from ICU, even when weaning or discharge protocols were used. Finally, the shorter time to extubation failed to translate into shorter time to ICU discharge in the two comparisons in the Canadian study [8]. One explanation for this difference may be low bed availability on the general wards. Another explanation may be the ongoing need for high level care immediately following early extubation.

Convincing evidence that the implementation of a sedation algorithm reduces the duration of mechanical ventilation and ICU stay has been provided by two propective, randomized, controlled trials [9, 10]. Furthermore, because caregivers might be likely to apply some sedation algorithm elements to non-algorithm patients enrolled in a randomized trial, the before-after sequential design used in the other controlled studies may be also considered appropriate. All these studies except one also showed a significant reduction in duration of mechancial ventilation in the algorithm-based sedation group. However, the imperative search for reduction in sedatives doses and duration of mechanical ventilation raises the question of the effect of these protocols on patient comfort and tolerance to the ICU environment during mechanical ventilation, which were not measured in most studies. Of note, no studies assessing selected outcomes in patients with non-invasive mechanical ventilation were identified.

Few studies have compared the benefit on the selected outcomes of intermittent "as needed" bolus doses vs continuous IV administration of neuromuscular blockers in the ICU. Despite a trend toward less persistent severe muscle weaknesses in the bolus group identified in one study, the small sample size, the exclusion of patients with renal failure, and methodological problems acknowledged by the authors may have masked the benefit of bolus vs continuous IV [13]. Furthermore, the effect on weaning time was not assessed. Although TOF monitoring has been largely advocated in recent consensus guidelines [3], only one prospective interventional study has shown that this has a positive effect on clinical outcome [14]. Although time to spontaneous ventilation was shorter, the clinical relevance of the benefit (2 hours) is uncertain. Nevertheless, in this study, greater (although not quantified) benefit on time to extubation was observed in patients with renal failure or concomitant administration of corticosteroids or aminoglycosides.

In conclusion, the use of specific sedative drugs and algorithms significantly reduces duration of mechanical ventilation or time to extubation after drug discontinuation. The precise benefit for patients receiving propofol in terms of duration of ICU or hospital stay, and the extent to which sedation algorithms adequately maintain patient comfort and tolerance to the ICU environment during mechanical ventilation warrants further investigation. To date, the benefit of a specific neuromuscular blocking drug or strategy has not been demonstrated.

References

1. Hansen-Flaschen JH, Brazinsky S, Basile C, Lanken PN (1991) Use of sedating drugs and neuromuscular blocking agents in patients requiring mechanical ventilation for respiratory failure. A national survey. JAMA 266:2870-2875
2. Jacobi J, Fraser GL, Coursin DB, et al (2002) Clinical practice guidelines for the sustained use of sedatives and analgesics in the critically ill adult. Crit Care Med 30:119-141
3. Murray MJ, Cowen J, DeBlock H, et al (2002) Clinical practice guidelines for sustained neuromuscular blockade in the adult critically ill patient. Crit Care Med 30:142-156
4. Garnacho-Montero J, Madrazo-Osuna J, Garcia-Garmendia JL, et al (2001) Critical illness polyneuropathy: risk factors and clinical consequences. A cohort study in septic patients. Intensive Care Med 27:1288-1296
5. Walder B, Elia N, Henzi I, Romand JR, Tramer MR (2001) A lack of evidence of superiority of propofol versus midazolam for sedation in mechanically ventilated critically ill patients: a qualitative and quantitative systematic review. Anesth Analg 92:975-983
6. Carrasco G, Molina R, Costa J, Soler JM, Cabre L (1993) Propofol vs midazolam in short-, medium-, and long-term sedation of critically ill patients. A cost-benefit analysis. Chest 103:557-564
7. Barrientos-Vega R, Mar Sanchez-Soria M, Morales-Garcia C, Robas-Gomez A, Cuena-Boy R, Ayensa-Rincon A (1997) Prolonged sedation of critically ill patients with midazolam or propofol: impact on weaning and costs. Crit Care Med 25:33-40
8. Hall RI, Sandham D, Cardinal P, et al (2001) Propofol vs midazolam for ICU sedation : a Canadian multicenter randomized trial. Chest 119:1151-1159
9. Brook AD, Ahrens TS, Schaiff R, et al (1999) Effect of a nursing-implemented sedation protocol on the duration of mechanical ventilation. Crit Care Med 27:2609-2615
10. Kress J, Pohlman A, O'Connor M, Hall J (2000) Daily interruption of sedative infusions in critically ill patients undergoing mechanical ventilation . N Engl J Med 342: 1471-1477
11. MacLaren R, Plamondon JM, Ramsay KB, Rocker GM, Patrick WD, Hall RI (2000) A prospective evaluation of empiric versus protocol-based sedation and analgesia. Pharmacotherapy 20:662-672
12. Brattebo G, Hofoss D, Flaatten H, Muri AK, Gjerde S, Plsek PE (2002) Effect of a scoring system and protocol for sedation on duration of patients' need for ventilator support in a surgical intensive care unit. Br Med J 324:1386-1389
13. de Lemos JM, Carr RR, Shalansky KF, Bevan DR, Ronco JJ (1999) Paralysis in the critically ill: intermittent bolus pancuronium compared with continuous infusion. Crit Care Med 27:2648-2655
14. Rudis MI, Sikora CA, Angus E, et al (1997) A prospective, randomized, controlled evaluation of peripheral nerve stimulation versus standard clinical dosing of neuromuscular blocking agents in critically ill patients. Crit Care Med 25:575-583
15. Strange C, Vaughan L, Franklin C, Johnson J (1997) Comparison of train-of-four and best clinical assessment during continuous paralysis. Am J Respir Crit Care Med 156:1556-1561
16. Mascia MF, Koch M, Medicis JJ (2000) Pharmacoeconomic impact of rational use guidelines on the provision of analgesia, sedation, and neuromuscular blockade in critical care. Crit Care Med 28:2300-2306
17. Ostermann ME, Keenan SP, Seiferling RA, Sibbald WJ (2000) Sedation in the intensive care unit: a systematic review. JAMA 283:1451-1459

Current Clinical Trials in Acute Lung Injury

M. O. Meade, K. E. Burns, and N. Adhikari

Introduction

Acute lung injury (ALI) is one of the most challenging syndromes that critical care clinicians encounter. A common complication of many critical illnesses, ALI affects all age groups and has a high associated mortality (30–70%). Not one of more than 20 tested drugs has been shown to improve survival. However, a recent pivotal study of a lung-protective ventilation strategy, using tidal volumes of 6 ml/kg predicted body weight has changed clinicians goals for supportive care, improved patient survival, and set a new standard for clinical research in this field [1]. With renewed enthusiasm, clinical investigators are evaluating a broad range of ALI interventions in large, collaborative randomized trials.

The aim of this brief chapter is to highlight the methodological and clinical importance of clinical trials currently underway in the field of ALI.

Methods

We consulted four databases (MEDLINE, EMBASE, the Cochrane Database of Systematic Reviews; from 1999 to 2002), three web sites (www.controlled-trials.com, www.clinicaltrials.gov, and www.ardsnet.org), abstracts published in four journals (*Intensive Care Medicine*, *Critical Care Medicine*, the *American Journal of Respiratory and Critical Care Medicine* and *Chest*), and ALI investigators for information related to ongoing randomized controlled trials designed to assess the effects of interventions on survival of patients with ALI. Our objective was to describe research methods and the current status of these trials rather than preliminary results.

Open Lung Ventilation

The goal of open lung ventilation is to minimize alveolar collapse, and thereby to improve gas exchange and protect the lungs from ventilator-associated injury related to shearing, overdistention, and oxygen toxicity. In a small multicenter trial, Brazilian investigators were the first to test an innovative strategy that combined: i) lung recruitment maneuvers (to open collapsed lung units), ii) liberal positive end-expiratory pressure (PEEP; to maintain alveolar recruitment), and iii) tidal volume limitation at 6 ml/kg [2]. Their findings included a statistically significant reduction in 28-day mortality (relative risk [RR] 0.53; 95% confidence interval [CI] 0.31–0.91) for patients with acute respiratory dictress syndrome (ARDS). However, the small difference in the number of events between control (17/24) and experimental (11/29) patients, a mere difference of six deaths, limits the applicability of these results to clinical practice.

To clarify the role for open lung ventilation in standard practice, three additional randomized controlled trials are underway.

"ALVEOLI" is a trial of the ARDS Network (www.ardsnet.org) that compares a high PEEP/low tidal volume strategy to a low PEEP/low tidal volume strategy among patients across the spectrum of ALI severity. Investigators concealed allocation, balanced potentially important cointerventions between the groups, employed a weaning protocol, achieved 100% follow-up, and conducted an intention-to-treat analysis. This study recently stopped prematurely (N=550) for lack of apparent efficacy; however, results related to pulmonary physiology, morbidity and mortality have not yet been published.

Well underway in 23 centres across Canada, the "Lung Open Ventilation Study" is a another trial including patients with moderately severe ALI (PaO_2/FiO_2 less than 250) [3]. The experimental ventilation strategy includes pressure control mode, tidal volumes of 6 ml/kg predicted body weight, plateau airway pressures not exceeding 40 cmH_2O, a liberal PEEP strategy, and lung recruitment maneuvers following ventilator disconnects. Protocols for adjusting PEEP and inspired oxygen according to arterial oxygenation result in significantly higher PEEP levels in the experimental group than the control group. The control strategy utilizes the 6 ml/kg tidal volume strategy shown to save lives [1]. Patients in both groups undergo a daily assessment for a trial of unassisted breathing. To date, nearly half of the target 980 patients have been randomized.

A related study underway in 45 centres across France is the "EXPRESS" trial. Eight hundred and fifty patients with ALI will receive tidal volume limitation (6 ml/kg) and only PEEP levels vary between the two groups. PEEP titration in the two groups is quite distinct from other trials: for control patients, total PEEP levels range from 5 to 9 cmH_2O while in the experimental strategy, PEEP is adjusted to maintain plateau airway pressure between 28 and 30 cmH_2O.

Ultimately, these four trials enrolling nearly 2,500 patients should resolve the role for liberal PEEP in ALI with respect to patient important outcomes. They may help to clarify an optimal threshold for plateau airway pressure. These trials are also likely to advance understanding of the pathophysiology of mechanical ventilation in ALI and provide data on the safety of lung recruitment maneuvers.

Prone Ventilation

The goal of prone positioning is to improve matching of ventilation and perfusion, and thereby improve oxygenation and survival. However, the potential for such serious complications as inadvertent extubation, loss of central venous access and chest tubes, delayed cardiopulmonary resuscitation, and blindness, is concerning.

In addition, a published multicenter, randomized controlled trial failed to show a survival benefit when patients with ALI or ARDS were nursed in the prone position for a minimum of 6 hours daily [4]. Investigators did observe, however, improved oxygenation and evolution of ALI, particularly for patients with more severe lung injury. In an intriguing post hoc analysis these patients were found to derive a non-statistically significant survival benefit.

Two multicenter randomized trials are underway in Spain and France. The Spanish trial has randomized more than 130 patients with ARDS. In this study, patients are ventilated in the prone position for 20 hours per day, significantly longer than in the prior trial. All patients are ventilated using assist control mode and weaned using pressure support. The primary endpoint in this trial is ICU mortality. In contrast, the French trial includes patients across the spectrum of severity of ALI and includes prone ventilation for a minimum of 8 hours per day. This study is approaching the planned sample size of 760 patients [5].

Inhaled Nitric Oxide

Inhaled nitric oxide (NO) is a selective pulmonary vasodilator that improves blood flow to ventilated regions of the lung. An acute improvement in oxygenation is apparent among 65% of patients; therefore, inhaled NO is used both for patients in respiratory *extremis* and to reduce inspired oxygen concentration among patients with perceived risk of oxygen toxicity. Inhaled NO is also used to decrease pulmonary artery pressure.

Among four published RCTs including 428 patients [6–9], features of design, population, and intervention were variable. Two studies were concealed [6, 7], one was blinded [6] one included only patients with severe ARDS (PaO_2/FiO_2 less than 150) [8], and one large trial included only patients who were identified as "NO-responders". NO doses and delivery methods varied across studies. Crossovers were rare, all studies achieved 100% follow-up and all included an intention-to-treat analysis. While one trial showed no effect of inhaled NO on survival [6], three others showed a trend toward increased mortality, raising concerns about the safety of inhaled NO. A systematic review and meta-analysis of published trials of NO for acute hypoxemic respiratory failure in adults and children showed no effect on survival [10].

Two additional multicenter trials hav not yet been published. A trial in France randomly assigned 203 ALI patients from 27 centres to 10 parts per million (ppm) inhaled NO or to placebo and reported preliminary data showing no effect on the evolution of ARDS, duration of mechanical ventilation, or mortality at 28 days [11]. An American trial enrolled 385 patients, with PaO_2/FiO_2 less than 250 and no significant non-respiratory organ failure, to receive 5 ppm of inhaled NO or placebo [12]. If the results of these trials are consistent with earlier randomized controlled trials, inhaled NO therapy in ALI may be restricted to the management of pulmonary hypertension or as a rescue therapy for life-threatening hypoxemia.

Extracorporeal Membrane Oxygenation (ECMO)

ECMO is an invasive intervention designed to rest the lungs and augment gas exchange with the use of cardiopulmonary bypass technology. Although two small randomized controlled trials found no effect on mortality [13, 14], ECMO methods in early trials bear little resemblance to present-day procedures, limiting their relevance to contemporary management of ALI.

In the current "CESAR" trial (www.cesar-trial.org), 67 centres in the UK have united to investigate ECMO among adults with severe ARDS, defined by severe hypoxemia or uncompensated hypercapnia. A study transport team transfers all patients assigned to ECMO therapy to a single ECMO centre. ECMO technology includes a veno-venous circuit with a high flow extracorporeal membrane. To achieve lung rest during ECMO therapy, patients are ventilated using peak inspiratory pressures up to 20 cmH$_2$O, PEEP 10 cmH$_2$O, respiratory rate 10 breaths per minute, and 30% FiO$_2$. For all control group patients, ventilation according to the US 6 ml/kg strategy is recommended; however, physicians are permitted to manage control patients at their discretion, with complete documentation of additional experimental respiratory interventions. Since the launch of this trial in April 2001, 69 of the target 240 patients have been enrolled. Investigators are planning intention-to-treat analyses of death and disability at 6 months after randomization, as well as an economic evaluation.

Pulmonary Arterial Catheters, Fluid Management, and Corticosteroids

The ARDS Network has two additional trials in progress. The "FACCT" trial is a 2 by 2 factorial design RCT comparing: i) a conservative versus a liberal fluid management strategy, and ii) monitoring with pulmonary arterial catheters versus central venous catheters among 1000 patients with ALI and ARDS. The placebo-controlled "Late Steroid Rescue Study" tests the hypothesis that systemic corticosteroids may prevent fibroproliferation in severe, late phase ARDS, thus improving gas exchange, lung compliance and patient survival. Although the original goal was to randomize 400 patients in this trial, the present target is 180 patients, over 3/4 of whom have been enrolled. Both studies employ tidal volume limitation (6 ml/kg) and a weaning protocol. The primary outcome in each of these trials is 60-day mortality; secondary outcomes include ventilator free days and organ failure free days.

Surfactant Therapy

Lung surfactant deficiency and dysfunction among patients with ARDS may contribute to abnormalities of gas exchange and lung compliance, and increase susceptibility to ventilator-associated lung injury. Results of seven randomized controlled trials enrolling 1352 patients suggest that there may be a role for surfactant therapy among adults with ALI [15] although results of the larger and more rigorous trials were less promising. Early trials included a variety of surfactant preparations (synthetic and animal surfactants) that varied in surfactant protein content, several methods of delivery (continuous or intermittent aerosolization; intratracheal instillation), and different dosages. In aggregate, too few patients have been studied to date to reliably assess the effect of surfactant on survival.

There are now several randomized controlled trials of surfactant therapies in progress or awaiting publication. Current randomized controlled trials in North America, Europe, and South Africa utilize tracheal administration of recombinant surfactant protein or calf lung surfactant, and employ low tidal volume ventilation and weaning protocols.

Miscellaneous

There are, additionally, large multicenter, placebo-controlled, industry-sponsored trials underway in Europe and North America evaluating the role for several intravenous therapies for patients with ALI. These drugs include, but are not limited to, a neutrophil elastase inhibitor (Sivelestat), and recombinant human atrial natriuretic peptide (Carperitide).

Conclusion

Current trials in ALI are investigating a broad range of interventions for the management of patients with ALI. We found a number of ongoing trials evaluating lung-protective ventilation strategies, other adjunctive respiratory support strategies, fluid management strategies, monitoring strategies, systemic corticosteroids, and novel pharmacologic therapies. These trials are of sufficient size and rigor that results may alter clinical practice in important ways. Relatively new intravenous therapies are also under investigation.

The prevalence of large, multicenter, collaborative trials reflects a trend in critical care research toward large studies to answer questions related to patient important outcomes rather than smaller studies evaluating primarily physiologic outcomes [16]. Several ongoing trials include ICU-, hospital-, and 6 month mortality; duration of ventilation, ICU care and hospitalization; organ dysfunction in the ICU; long term morbidity and health related quality of life; and cost effectiveness outcomes. The inclusion of large numbers of patients provides a unique opportunity to systematically collect a range of data to improve our understanding of disease as well as clinical management. This is also an advantage to multiple trials testing closely related interventions [17].

We also found that current trials incorporate significant clinical findings and methodological advances of earlier trials. To prevent selection bias, randomization is concealed. To address potential intervention bias, investigators standardize ventilation protocols using 6 ml/kg (where applicable, just for control patients) and generally include weaning protocols, which have been shown to reduce the duration of ventilation and may influence patient outcomes [18].

In summary, ALI is an extremely active field of clinical research. Current clinical trials are large, rigorous and more likely than ever before to influence the care of critically ill patients with ALI.

References

1. The Acute Respiratory Distress Syndrome Network (2000) Ventilation with lower tidal volumes as compared with traditional tidal volumes for acute lung injury and the acute respiratory distress syndrome.. N Engl J Med 342:1301–1308
2. Amato MB, Barbas CS, Medeiros DM, et al (1998) Effect of a protective ventilation strategy on mortality in the acute respiratory distress syndrome. N Engl J Med 338:347–354
3. Meade MO, Stewart TE, Guyatt GH, et al (2002) Adherence to protocol in an acute lung injury management trial. Am J Respir Crit Care Med 165:A27 (abst)
4. Gattinoni L, Tognoni G, Pesenti A, et al., for the Prone-Supine Study Group (2001) Effect of prone positioning on the survival of patients with acute respiratory failure. N Engl J Med 345:568–573
5. Gaillard S, Guerin C (2001) A multicenter randomized trail of early prone positioning of patients with acute respiratory failure: interim analysis. Am J Respir Crit Care Med 163:A16 (abst)
6. Dellinger RP, Zimmerman JL, Taylor RW, et al (1998) Effects of inhaled nitric oxide in patients with acute respiratory distress syndrome: Results of a randomized phase II trial. Crit Care Med 26:15–23
7. Lundin S, Mang H, Smithies M, Stenqvist O, Frostell C, for the European Study Group of Inhaled Nitric Oxide (1999) Intensive Care Med 25:911–919
8. Michael JR, Barton RG, Saffle JR, et al (1998) Inhaled nitric oxide versus conventional therapy. Effect on oxygenation in ARDS. Am J Respir Crit Care Med 157:1372–1380
9. Troncy E, Collet JP, Shapiro S, et al (1998) Inhaled nitric oxide in acute respiratory distress syndrome. A pilot randomized controlled study. Am J Respir Crit Care Med 157:1483–1488
10. Sokol J, Jacobs SE, Bohn D (2000) Inhaled nitric oxide for acute respiratory failure in children and adults. Cochrane Database Syst Rev CD002787
11. Payen D, Vallet B, and the Groupe dEtude du NO dans lARDS (1999) Results of the French prospective multicentre randomized double-blind placebo-controlled trial in inhaled nitric oxide (NO) in ARDS. Intensive Care Med 25:A645 (abst)
12. Wood KA, Linde-Zwirble WT, Clermont G, et al (2002) Am J Respir Crit Care Med 165:A220 (abst)
13. Zapol WM, Snider MT, Hill JD, et al (1979) Extracorporeal membrane oxygenation in severe acute respiratory failure. A randomized prospective study. JAMA 242:2193–2196
14. Morris AH, Wallace CJ, Menlove RL, et al (1994) Randomized clinical trial of pressure-controlled inverse ratio ventilation and extracorporeal CO_2 removal for adult respiratory distress syndrome. Am J Respir Crit Care Med 149:295–305
15. Adhikari N, Burns K, Meade MO (2003) A systematic review of pharmacologic therapies for the acute respiratory distress syndrome and acute lung injury. Am J Respir Med (in press)
16. Graf J, Doig GS, Cook DJ, Vincent JL, Sibbald WJ (2002) Randomized, controlled clinical trials in sepsis: has methodologic quality improved over time? Crit Care Med 30:461–472
17. Hebert PC, Cook DJ, Wells G, Marshall J (2002) The design of randomized clinical trials in critically ill patients. Chest 121:1290–1300
18. Ely EW, Baker AM, Dunagan DP, et al (1996) Effect on the duration of mechanical ventilation of identifying patients capable of breathing spontaneously. N Engl J Med 335:1864–1869

Novel Advancements in the Management and Diagnosis of Acute Respiratory Failure

C. C. dos Santos and A. S. Slutsky

Introduction

Over the past decade, patients with acute respiratory failure have benefited more from scientific advancements than in the preceding three decades. Important knowledge has enabled the reduction in the expected mortality from ARDS from well over 50% [1] to as low as 30% [2, 3]. Much of this advancement has come from recognition of the impact of iatrogenic complications related to the stay in the intensive care unit (ICU). The advent of basic prevention strategies for critically ill patients – from elevation of the head of the bed for prevention of ventilator associated pneumonia (VAP) [4] to the use of low molecular weight heparin for the prevention of deep vein thrombosis (DVT) [5, 6]- has provided intensivists with the tools to reduce morbidity and mortality in this patient population. In the field of acute lung injury (ALI), evidence indicates that reducing tidal volume during mechanical ventilation reduces mortality by over 20% [7].

Despite advances in the management of the critical care patient, much of what we have learned relates to what therapies do not work and why they do not work; we are still struggling to try and develop a fundamental breakthrough in ALI. The future holds great promise however. There are two main reasons for this optimism: (1) a community of health care providers that is multi-disciplinary in nature and diverse in scope and interest is coming together, with the common goal of advancing knowledge and professional care in this particular field; (2) the advent of sophisticated tools to answer more fundamental questions. Important advancements in the fields of molecular genetics and immunology, bioinformatics and bioengineering are being developed. Consequently this is a uniquely exciting and challenging time to be involved in critical care research and clinical practice. This chapter will focus on some novel approaches that are currently being developed and may have a clinical impact in the next few years for the diagnosis and management of patients with acute respiratory failure.

Neural Control of Ventilation

Poor coupling between the patient and the ventilator remains one of the main problems in the management of patients with acute respiratory failure, especially those with obstructive lung diseases. For the most part, if the ventilator and the patient's respiratory cycles are not matched, the patient tends to 'resist' the ventilator, causing discomfort, gas exchange deterioration, and cardiovascular impairment. One common approach that is used clinically to increase coordination between the patient and the ventilator is to change the patient's drive by overventilation [8], increasing sedation [9] and/or pharmacologic paralysis [10]. These approaches are associated with numerous complications. A more appealing approach is to make the ventilation more responsive to the patient's ventilatory demands. At present, airway pressure, flow or volume is used to initiate and regulate the ventilator in assisted forms of ventilation. This approach is effective in patients with relatively normal lungs where the changes in flow and pressure at the airway opening occur almost coincident with the patient's ventilatory demands (i.e., neural output from the brain stem). However, in many patients there are important delays between neural activation and pressure/flow generation at the airway opening.

In patients with chronic obstructive pulmonary disease (COPD), severe expiratory flow limitation leads to gas trapping and an increase in intra-thoracic pressure (intrinsic positive end expiratory pressure or auto-PEEP) [11]. Auto-PEEP must be overcome before negative intra-thoracic pressure or flow can be generated to trigger the ventilator. This imposes an additional load on the respiratory muscles [12, 13]. Although auto-PEEP can be counter-balanced by the use of extrinsic PEEP [14], the difficulty in clinically determining intrinsic PEEP makes the determination of the appropriate extrinsic PEEP a matter of trial and error. The application of excessive external PEEP also has its complications, such as causing further hyperinflation [15], adding to the impairment of the diaphragm [16], failing hemodynamics and gas exchange, and increased risk of barotrauma [17].

The ideal approach to coordinate mechanical assistance with patient demands would be to control the timing and the magnitude of positive pressure applied by the ventilator. Direct measurement of the output of the respiratory center for this purpose is not feasible at present. Transforming neural drive into ventilatory output (neuro-ventilatory-coupling) can be achieved using measurements of neuronal excitation of the diaphragm [18]. Recent technological advances have made it possible for reliable signals from the diaphragm to be obtained, free from artifacts and noise from the heart and esophagus [19]. Diaphragmatic electrical activity can also provide a means to give continuous ventilatory assist in proportion to the neural drive, both within a given breath and between breaths – a technique known as neurally adjusted ventilatory assist (NAVA) [13]. With NAVA, the

Fig. 1. a. Steps necessary to transform central respiratory drive into an inspiration. **b.** Impaired patient-ventilator interaction during airway pressure triggered ventilatory assist. Delay from onset of inspiratory effort, indicated by the beginning of diaphragmatic electrical activity (vertical lines) and the negative deflection in esophageal pressure, to start ventilator mechanical assistance. Wasted efforts are demonstrated. **c.** Electrode array arrangement. (i) attached to the nasogastric tube. The electrode array is positioned perpendicular to the crural diaphragm. Signals from the each electrode pair is differentially amplified, (iii) digitized into a personal computer, and (iv) filtered to remove the noise. The processed signal's intensity value is displayed on the monitor or fed to the ventilator (v). From [13] with permission

Novel Advancements in the Management and Diagnosis of Acute Respiratory Failure   151

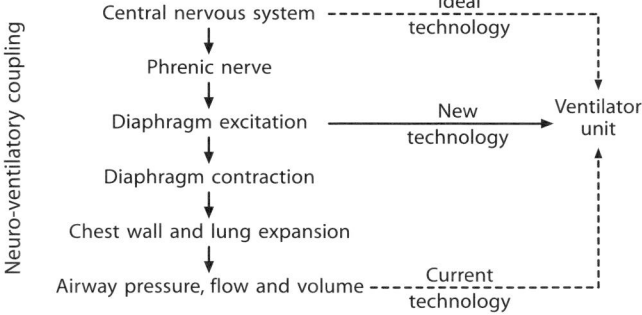

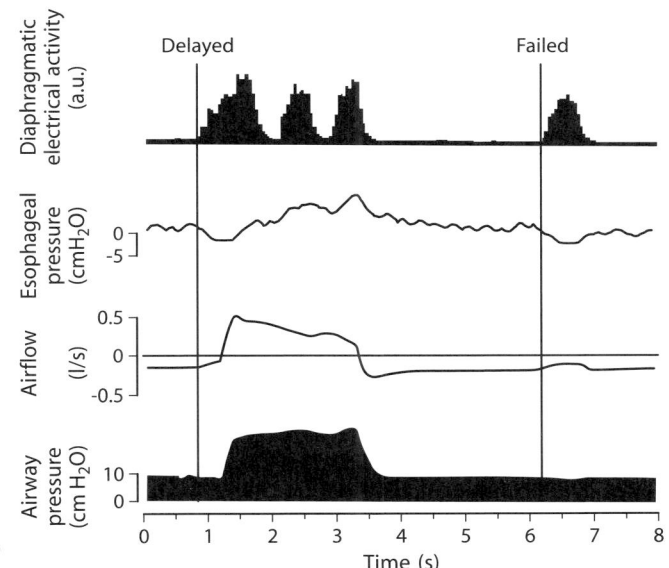

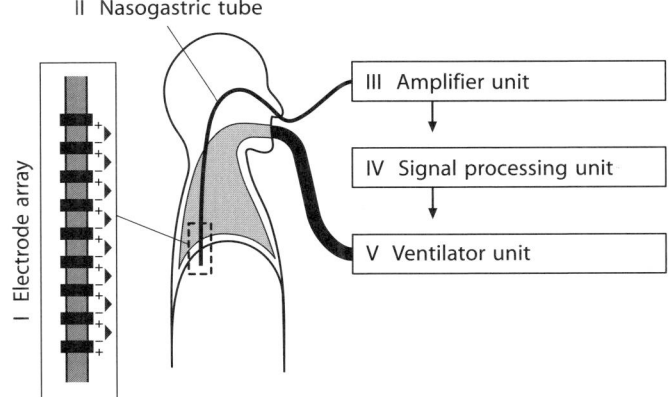

Fig. 2. a. Conventional pressure trigger: Mechanical assistance starts when airway pressure decreases. The beginning of inspiratory effort (solid vertical lines) precedes inspiratory flow. Further delay occurs from the onset of inspiratory flow (dashed vertical lines) to the rise in positive airway pressure, due to the mechanical limitations of the ventilator trigger. **b.** Neural triggering: The ventilator provides support as soon as diaphragmatic electrical activity exceeds a threshold value. The delay to onset of inspiratory flow and increased airway pressure is almost eliminated. **c.** Diaphragmatic electrical activity (shaded areas) is poorly coordinated with the ventilatory support, and often results in wasted inspiratory efforts. **d.** Implementation of neural trigger can restore the interaction between the patient's neural drive and the ventilatory support. From [13] with permission

magnitude of the mechanical support varies according to a mathematical function that represents the diaphragmatic electrical activity multiplied by a gain factor selected on the machine. This allows for the patient's respiratory center to be in control of the mechanical support provided throughout the course of each breath, allowing any variation in neural respiratory output to be matched by a corresponding change in ventilatory assistance.

Sinderby et al. have described an automated method for on-line acquisition and processing of diaphragmatic electrical signals that represent the neuronal drive to the diaphragm [13, 20]. This system relies on bipolar electrodes positioned in the lower esophagus (electrode array can be placed along the distal portion of the nasogastric or orogastric tube) to measure diaphragmatic electrical activity. Signals from each electrode pair are differentially amplified, digitized, and processed using filters that give the highest signal-to-noise ratio. This allows for the determination of the position of the electrically active region of the activated diaphragm (EARdi). Because the electrodes are arranged in a perpendicular array, all signals are obtained in phase. Signals on the opposite side of the EARdi correlate with extreme negative values, versus signals of the same side of the EARdi that correlate with extreme positive values. Signal segments with residual disturbance from cardiac electrical activity can be eliminated via the use of specific filters. The final signal, with enhanced signal-to-noise ratio, can then be transferred to the ventilator unit for monitoring and regulation of the ventilatory assist [21, 22]. Finally signals can be fed to the ventilatory assist for the execution of NAVA (see Figs 1, 2 and 3 for details).

The electrical activity recorded from a muscle constitutes the spatial and temporal summation of action potential from the recruited motor units. Some of the relevant factors that influence neuro-mechanical coupling include both dynamic and static changes in lung volume [20, 23]. Recently Sinderby et al. demonstrated that esophageal recordings of crural EARdi can be used to determine changes in global diaphragm activation (i.e., respiratory drive) in a group of mechanically ventilated patients with acute respiratory failure [20, 24]. This was obtained when no evidence for changes in neuro-mechanical coupling were found (with varying levels of pressure support). The use of esophageal recordings to evaluate diaphragm activation in acute respiratory failure is most often criticized because of claims that the signal strength is affected by changes in lung volume. In this recent paper, however, this group demonstrated that the measurements of diaphragmatic

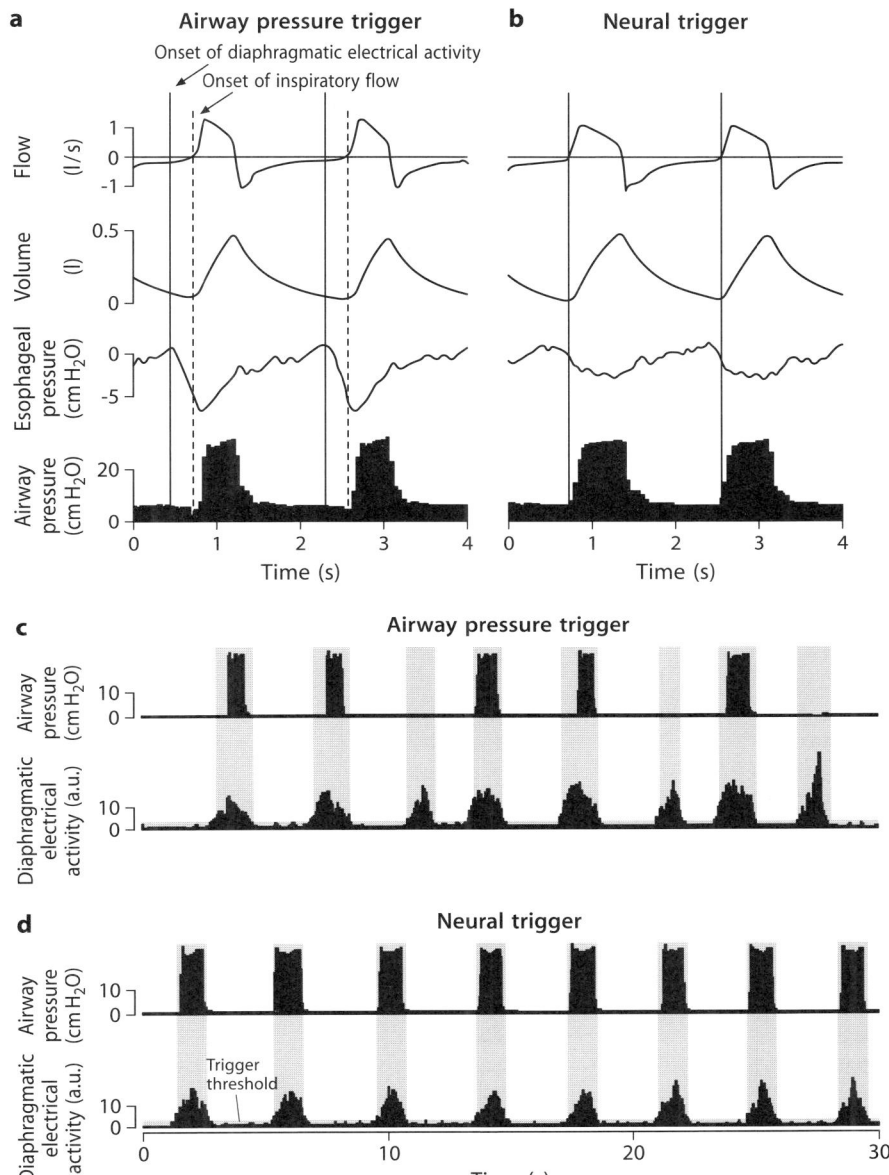

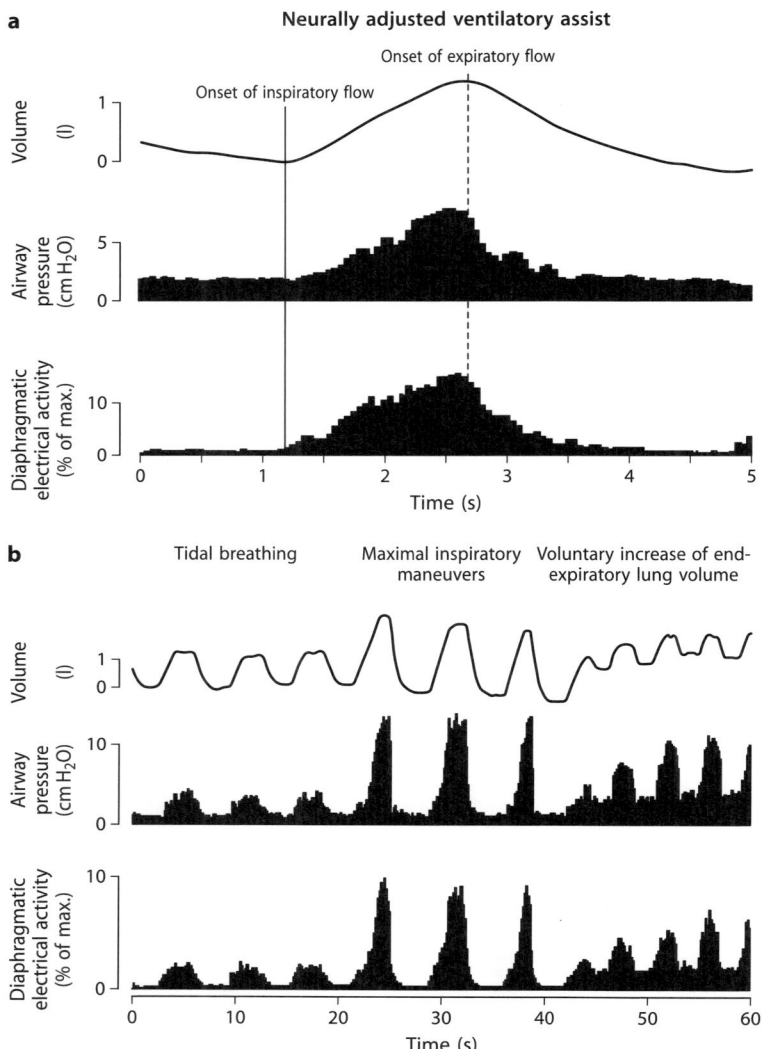

Fig.3. Neurally adjusted ventilatory assist. **a.** Neurally adjusted ventilatory assist during a single breath during various breathing maneuvers. **b.** There is continuous proportional adjustment of airway pressure (reflecting ventilatory assist) with changes in diaphragmatic electrical activity (reflecting neural drive) during changes in tidal and end-expiratory lung volumes. From [13] with permission

electrical activity are not artifactually influenced by changes in chest wall configuration and/or lung volume during voluntary contraction [25]. In addition, any increase in diaphragmatic electrical activity observed with an increase in lung volume, represents a true increase in neural drive to the diaphragm that is required to compensate for the shortened length [25]. This method has been validated in healthy subjects during both static [2] and dynamic [3] maneuvers, as well as in patients with diaphragm weakness (caused by chronic obstructive lung disease or polio), at rest [4] and during exercise [26].

Many patient groups should benefit from the use of neuronal triggering and NAVA, as long as the respiratory center, phrenic nerve, and neuromuscular junction are intact. Contraindications that preclude electrode catheter placement may be another limitation to the use of this technology. In addition, the use of diaphragmatic electrical activity to estimate respiratory center output assumes the diaphragm to be the primary inspiratory muscle. In the future, randomized clinical trials are required to determine if the use of neural control of ventilation strategies will improve important outcomes in the management of the ALI patient.

Electrical Impedance Tomography

Part of the difficulty in developing effective therapies for acute respiratory distress syndrome (ARDS) is the heterogeneous nature of the disease and its complex pathophysiology. We know from a number of studies that overdistention of lung units, and allowing the lung to repetitively undergo cyclic recruitment/de-recruitment, can lead to various forms of lung injury termed barotrauma, volutrauma, atelectrauma and biotrauma [26-28].

The key to mitigating these types of injury is to recruit lung units, while at the same time minimizing overdistention - a task which is made particularly difficult because of the tremendous anatomic heterogeneity of the underlying disease process. Some approaches that have been used to accomplish this aim include use of pressure/volume (P/V) curves [29], use of a PEEP/FiO2 table [30, 31] and monitoring the shape of the pressure-time curve [32]. All of these approaches have some value, but ideally we would like to be able to visualize the entire lung to try and minimize the different forms of lung injury described above. Therein lies the advantage of electrical impedance tomography (EIT), a non-invasive, radiation free imaging technique that provides clinical information regarding regional lung structure.

EIT, also called applied potential tomography, is a novel imaging technique developed in the 1980s by Barber and Brown [33, 34]. EIT is based on the principle of measuring potential differences on the surface of the body, resulting from the application of repetitive small alternating electrical currents. This information is used to calculate the distribution of electrical impedance in the body cross-section that can be visually presented in the form of two-dimensional tomographs (Fig. 4). Compared with techniques such as computerized x-ray tomography and positron emission tomography, EIT is about a thousand times cheaper, a thousand times smaller, and requires no ionizing radiation. Further, EIT can in principle produce thousands of images per second. Recordings are typically made by applying current

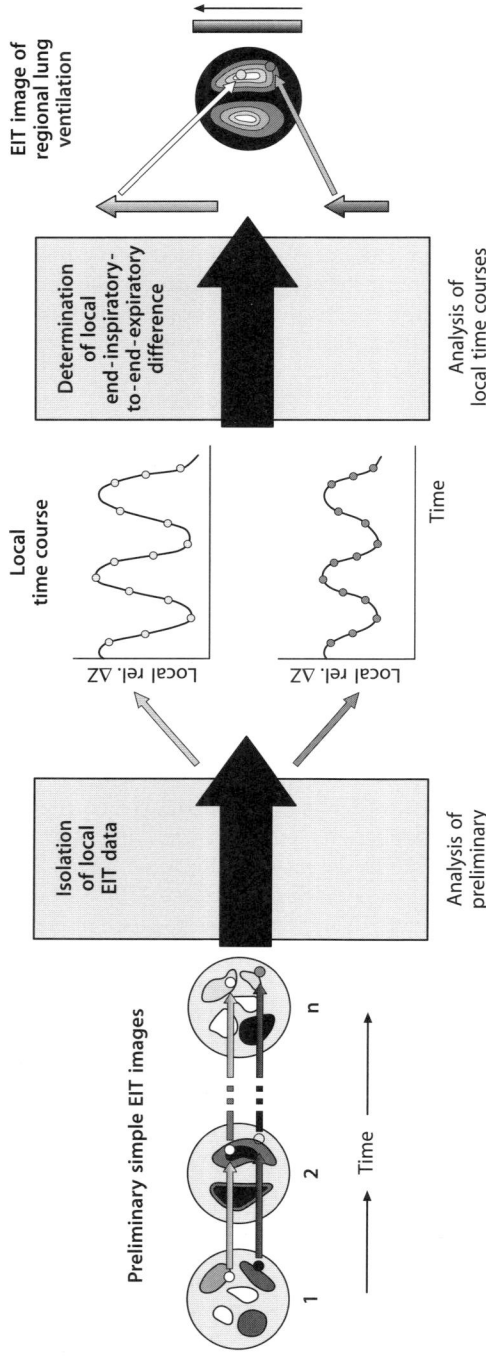

Fig.4. Generation of an electrical impedance tomography (EIT) image of regional lung ventilation from a sequence of preliminary simple EIT images originating from one EIT measurements. The image orientation is the following: dorsal at the top and the right side of the body is on the left of the image. From [77] with permission

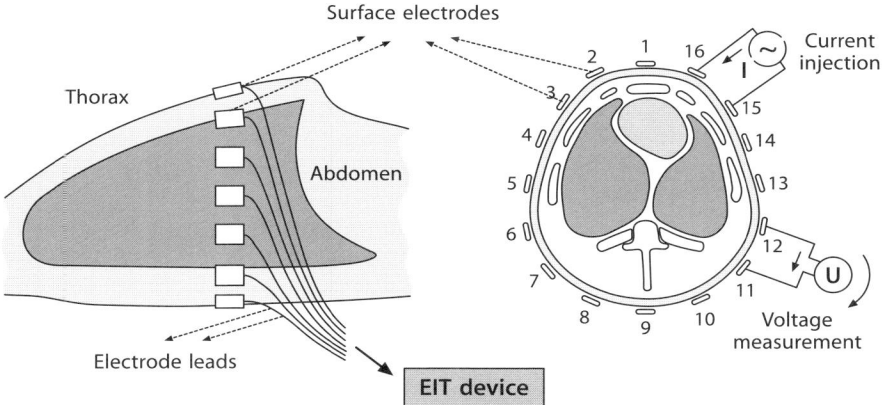

Fig. 5. Electrical excitation currents (I) are consecutively placed between pairs of adjacent surface electrodes after each current injection resulting voltages are measured From [78] with permission

to the body or system under test using a set of electrodes, and measuring the voltage developed between other electrodes (Figs 4, 5). To obtain reasonable images, at least one hundred, and preferably several thousand, such measurements must be made.

EIT produces images of the distribution of impedivity (or, more commonly, resistivity), or its variation with time or frequency, within the tissue. There is a large resistivity contrast (up to about 200:1) between a wide range of tissue types in the body [35, 36], making it possible to use resistivity to form anatomical images which can separate gas containing from non-gas containing regions (Fig. 5). To measure resistivity or impedivity, a current – referred to as the excitation current - must flow in the tissue and the resulting voltages be measured. In practice, almost all EIT systems use constant current sources, and measure voltage differences between adjacent pairs of electrodes. To obtain an image with good spatial resolution, a number of such measurements are required. From the set of measurements, an image reconstruction technique generates the tomographic image. Mathematically, the known quantities are the voltages and currents at certain points on the body; the unknown is the impedivity or resistivity within the body. Until recently, the change in resistivity was measured over time, and EIT images were inherently of physiological function. It is now possible to produce anatomical images using the same reconstruction technique, by imaging changes with frequency [37].

There are multiple potential clinical applications for EIT [33]. Determination of extravascular lung water and regional ventilation are two problems that pertain specifically to the ICU patient [38–41]. In ARDS, lung density increases from the ventral to the dorsal lung regions in the supine position and an increased amount of extravascular lung water causes compression atelectasis in the posterior part. Because EIT can visualize regional ventilation, differences in the ventilation-induced impedance changes occurring between the anterior part and posterior part of the lungs provides information about the extravascular lung water content [41].

Previous studies proved the ability of EIT to detect changes in regional lung volumes and end-expiratory lung volumes induced by variation of tidal volume and PEEP under experimental conditions [18, 42–44]. In clinical settings, the effects of PEEP and the ventilation chosen (conventional, assisted, spontaneous) can also be determined [43, 45, 46]. This may be useful in determining response to treatment (Fig. 3). EIT may be used to assess recruitment and derecruitment as well as to obtain regional P/V curves in ARDS patients [45, 47].

The major limitations of EIT are its low spatial resolution, and large variability of images between subjects [48, 49]. In the future, the use of modern high performance EIT devices which exhibit a higher signal/noise ratio, enabling free selection of electrical current frequency and guaranteeing undisturbed measurements in the noisy environment, will hopefully improve the quality of EIT and increase the clinical acceptance of this method.

Ventilogenomics

Molecular genetics research has, in a handful of years, invaded the field of critical care medicine. What was difficult and complex research just a few years ago is now routine for most laboratories. In the field of ARDS, advances in molecular and medical genetics are expected to affect every aspect of this syndrome - from diagnosis and prevention to treatment and follow-up. To date, most of the efforts have focused on: (i) diagnosis of ARDS and (ii) treatment of this syndrome. As mentioned previously, part of the problem with ARDS is its complex nature. Our current diagnostic criteria do not incorporate the two major hallmarks of the pathophysiology of ARDS - the increase in lung permeability and the inflammatory nature of the injury. The unknown relationship between clinical syndrome and pathophysiology creates problems when attempts are made to define specific treatments.

One approach that has been used in the past and will certainly be used in the future to dissect out the basic mechanisms of ALI, is the use of mutant, knock-out, and transgenic animal models. For example, by measuring survival time, protein and neutrophil concentrations in bronchoalveolar lavage (BAL) fluid, lung wet-to-dry ratio, and histology, Leikauf et al. found that the susceptibility to nickel sulfate induced acute lung injury could be inherited [50]. Genome-wide analysis indicated significant linkage on murine chromosome 6 - Aliq4. In other studies of genetic susceptibility [51], cDNA microarray analyses indicated several pathogenic responses during nickel-induced ALI, including marked macrophage activation. Macrophage activation is mediated, in part, via the receptor tyrosine kinase Ron. To address the role of Ron in ALI, the response of mice deficient in the cytoplasmic domain of Ron (Ron tk-/-) were assessed in response to nickel exposure. Ron tk-/- mice succumbed to nickel-induced ALI earlier, expressed larger, early increases in interleukin-6, monocyte chemoattractant protein-1, and macrophage inflammatory protein-2, displayed greater serum nitrite levels, and exhibited earlier onset of pulmonary pathology and augmented pulmonary tyrosine nitrosylation. Increases in cytokine expression and cellular nitration can lead to tissue damage and are consistent with the differences between genotypes in the early onset of pathology and mortality in Ron tk-/- mice. This suggests that the absence of Ron may be a marker for inhaled particle induced ALI.

Human studies of genetic susceptibility to critical care illness have been published and are currently under intense investigation. For example, a guanine to adenine transition at the +250 site within the lymphotoxin-alpha (LT-α), also known as the tumor necrosis factor (TNF)-β gene [52–54], has been associated with variability in TNF-α secretion after endotoxin and other stimuli exposure, with increased levels associated with the A allele in both sites. The presence of the A allele at the LT-α +250 polymorphic site is associated with higher mortality from septic shock, with the AA homozygotes being at highest risk [55]. Similar findings have been reported with the TNF-α-308 gene polymorphism [56], although this may not always be the case [57]. In an effort to expand these results to genetic susceptibility to lung injury Waterer al. [58] explored the genetic susceptibility patterns of patients with community acquired pneumonia to develop sepsis or type I respiratory failure (which this group defined as an O2 saturation on room air of < 90% with a normal PCO2). Interestingly they found that while the presence of the LT-α +250 genotype was associated with the greatest risk of septic shock, it was not associated with the development of type I respiratory failure. Consistent with the current understanding of the pathophysiology of sepsis and septic shock, studies have shown that the LT-α +250 genotype is associated with greater TNF-α secretion after a variety of stimuli, both in vitro [52, 53] and in vivo [55, 59].

The first report of a positive association of a candidate gene polymorphism with the incidence of and outcome from ARDS has recently been published by Marshall et al. [60]. This group demonstrated a marked increase in the frequency of the D allele of the angiotensin converting enzyme (ACE) gene in patients with ARDS when compared with other ICU patients (p=0.00008), coronary bypass artery bypass grafting patients (p=0.0009), and the general population (p=0.00004). Moreover, this genotype was significantly associated with mortality in the ARDS group (p<0.02). These data suggest a potential role for the rennin-angiotensin system in the pathogenesis of ARDS and implicate genetic factors in the development and progression of this syndrome. ACE is an important effector molecule in the regulation of vascular tone and cardiac function. Other functions include neuronal metabolism (enkephalins, neurotensin, and substance P), reproduction (gonadotrophin luteinizing hormone releasing hormone) and digestion (cholecystokinin) [61]. Alterations in the function of the ACE may also change metabolic processes regulated by bradykinin, angiotensin (AT) I and ATII. Epidemiological studies are required to determine if the D allele of the ACE gene can represent the first of a series of genetic markers that will be used in the future to identify population at risks and perhaps further delineate the diagnostic criteria for ARDS. One of the important limitations of the study relates to the fact that ACE levels were not measured; consequently the relationship between the gene product and the phenotype remains unclear.

Given the observation that mechanical ventilation can lead to release of cytokines (biotrauma) [27], given that this cytokine release can be modulated by ventilatory strategy [64, 65], given that there is a suggestion that there is a relationship between interleukin (IL)-6 and mortality in ARDS that is modulated by mechanical ventilation [7], and given that the cytokine response in any individual is likely genetically determined as described above, suggests that it may be possible to predict which patients are predisposed to biotrauma. This approach – which may be termed ventilogenomics – could have important consequences in the future management of ventilated patients by identifying those patients at high risk of developing biotrauma. In those patients at high risk for biotrauma the clinician may decide to institute more aggressive lung protective strategies and/or apply immunomodulatory strategies (see next section) earlier.

Immunomodulation

Although improved imaging techniques and better ventilatory strategies are likely to improve the future management of patients with ALI, there almost certainly will be a need for other non-ventilatory approaches to mitigate ventilator-induced injury because of the tremendous heterogeneity in the lung injury. As such, various groups have been exploring the use of different strategies to modulate the underlying inflammatory response in ARDS and the biotrauma caused by mechanical ventilation. Recently published papers have provided an overview of the rationale behind various immunomodulating strategies and the results from human trials with different immunomodulating agents in patients with ARDS (please see [62, 63] for details). Some of the major strategies reviewed in these papers include the use of corticosteroids, antioxidants, and arachidonic acid metabolites. Other therapies include factors that affect the coagulation cascade, inhaled therapies such as nitric oxide (NO), partial liquid ventilation, and immunonutrition. The use of mechanical ventilation is an important adjunct to immunomodulatory therapies in ARDS. This concept has been explored by various groups, and recently the ARDS Network Trial showed that a protective ventilatory strategy that used low tidal volumes could reduce mortality by over 20% [7]. This difference in mortality has been deemed to be related to the ability of a protective ventilatory strategy to attenuate the increase in cytokines which have been shown to be involved in the generation and the progression of ARDS and multi-organ failure syndrome [7, 64, 65].In contrast, anti-cytokine therapy, has not received as much attention for the treatment of ARDS. Most of the knowledge on the subject has been extrapolated from the failed human sepsis trials. Although it is beyond the scope of this paper to review and evaluate this body of literature, suffice it to say that this is inadequate, and it may have led to the delay in the development of this line of therapy for ARDS.

To investigate whether anti-cytokine therapy may have a relevant role in the treatment of ALI, a rabbit model of ventilator-induced lung injury (VILI) was used to examine the effect of recombinant IL-1 receptor antagonist (IL-1ra) [66]. Animals maintained under pentobarbital anesthesia were primed for injury by undergoing lung lavage with 22 ml/kg of saline and then ventilated for 8 h with either FiO_2 0.21 and normal pressures, or FiO_2 1.0 and high ventilator pressures. The animals exposed to hyperoxia/hyperventilation demonstrated a greater increase in lung lavage neutrophil counts and a higher histological injury score, as well as a faster decline in oxygenation compared to the control animals. A third group of rabbits received 800 micrograms of recombinant IL-1ra after lung lavage and prior to the exposure to FiO2 1.0 and high ventilator pressures. These animals had significantly lower concentrations of albumin and elastase and lower neutrophil counts in their lungs after the 8-hour ventilatory period compared to hyperoxia/hyperventilation rabbits. IL-1 blockade had no effect on the decline in dynamic compliance and oxygenation seen in saline-treated hyperoxic/hyperventilated rabbits [66]. In previous studies, Ulich et al. explored the role of IL-1 in lipopolysaccharide (LPS)-induced acute pneumonia by quantifying the acute inflammation occurring at 6 hours after the intra-tracheal injection of LPS as compared to the same time point after the intra-tracheal coinjection of LPS and IL-1ra. IL-1ra was found to inhibit LPS-induced acute inflammation (p = 0.0001) as measured by the number of neutrophils recovered in bronchoalveolar lavage (BAL). In this study, the LPS-induced emigration of neutrophils was inhibited by as much as 45% [67]. Moreover, systemic administration of recombinant human IL-1ra causes a rapid and sustained elevation of plasma IL-1ra levels and decreases the leak of intravascularly injected 125I-labeled albumin into lungs of rats given human recombinant interleukin-1 intra-tracheally [68].

Imai et al. [69] evaluated the protective effects of anti-TNF-α antibody (Ab) in saline-lavage lung injury in rabbits. After saline lung lavage, polyclonal anti-TNF-α Ab was intra-tracheally instilled. Animals were divided into a high-dose group (1mg/kg), a low-dose group (0.2 mg/kg), serum IgG fraction in the Ab control group, and saline in the saline control group. After instillation of the polyclonal anti-TNF-α, Ab animals were ventilated using a conventional strategy for 4 h. Pretreatment with intra-tracheal instillation of high and low doses of anti-TNF-α Ab improved oxygenation and respiratory compliance, reduced the infiltration of leukocytes, and ameliorated pathological findings. In a mouse model of cotton dust induced acute lung injury, mice pretreated with anti-TNA-α antiserum displayed a marked attenuation of the neutrophilic inflammation. Interestingly, in this study the level of TNF-α mRNA expression was not reduced, suggesting that this inhibition is not related to the induction of a feed back loop that leads to inhibition of novel TNF-α gene expression, but rather may affect the activation of the downstream effectors of TNF-α [70]. This may explain why arresting the drive for de novo gene expression (e.g., reducing the effects of mechanical stretch) may have had a greater clinical impact (ARDS Net Trial) than the anti-cytokine therapy (as it has been used to date). If the insult that drives the increased expression of cytokines (such as IL-1b and TNF-α) is persistent, then perhaps anti-cytokine therapies should be used as continuous infusions. Moreover, if the lung acts as an immunomodulatory organ driving the systemic immune response in ARDS patients who develop multi-organ failure syndrome, then perhaps local (pulmonary) continuous infusions of anti-cytokine therapy may exert its beneficial effect whilst protecting from negative systemic effects of anti-cytokine therapy. Nevertheless, as new information about the pathophysiology of ARDS becomes available, the question of how to immunomodulate the inflammatory response will continue to intrigue investigators and critical care providers alike.

Molecular genetics is also a potential therapeutic target for ARDS. In a recent study, Weiss et al. [71] administered a recombinant E1, E3 deleted adenovirus expressing the gene for heat shock protein-70 (HSP-70; AdHSP-70)) directly into the trachea of rats at the time of cecal ligation and perforation. Administration of

AdHSP-70 significantly attenuated interstitial and alveolar edema and protein exudation and dramatically decreased neutrophil accumulation, relative to control. Mortality due to cecal ligation was also dramatically reduced. Presumably the protective effects of HSP-70 are secondary to its broad-spectrum defense mechanism, effective in protecting cells against all types of injury. This may be related to its function as a molecular chaperone, maintaining and repairing intracellular proteins.

An alternative hypothesis is that HSP-70 itself interacts specifically with the innate immune system thus conferring resistance to acute lung injury. Recent studies have initiated a paradigm shift in the understanding of the function of HSP. It is now clear that HSP can and do exit mammalian cells, interact with cells of the immune system, and exert immunoregulatory effects. Exogenously added HSP-70 possesses potent cytokine activity, with the ability to bind with high affinity to the plasma membrane, elicit a rapid intracellular Ca2+ flux, activate nuclear factor-kappa B (NF-κB), and up-regulate the expression of pro-inflammatory cytokines in human monocytes(72-74). HSP70-induced proinflammatory cytokine production is mediated via the MyD88/IRAK/NF-κB signal transduction pathway and HSP-70 utilizes both Toll-like receptor (TLR)2 (receptor for Gram-positive bacteria) and TLR4 (receptor for Gram-negative bacteria) to transduce its proinflammatory signal in a CD14-dependent fashion [75]. HSP-70 induces IL-12 and endothelial cell-leukocyte adhesion molecule-1 (ELAM-1) promoters in macrophages. This is controlled by MyD88 and TNF-receptor associated factor (TRAF)6 [76]. The ability of this ubiquitous stress response protein to act as an isolated endogenous ligand able to activate the ancient Toll/IL-1 receptor signal pathway is in line with the "danger hypothesis" proposing that the innate immune system senses danger signals even if they originate from self. Moreover, linkage between the HSP70-2 A allele and the previously reported mortality-related homozygous genotype, TNFB2/B2, has been identified in patients suffering from severe sepsis.

Molecular genetics and immunology research is moving relentlessly fast and soon will become part of the armamentarium to be incorporated into broad clinical research and practice. Additional developments in the field of bioinformatics are also fueling this fire. The extent of the impact of this new technology on current medical practice is impossible to predict and imagine.

Conclusion

Over the last few decades, the discipline of intensive care has established itself with dedicated training schemes and practitioners. Over the next few years, intensivists will have to develop the skills to exploit novel tools originating from a variety of sources - from bioengineering to molecular biology - to improve the care of their critically ill patients. Moreover, the complex nature of acute respiratory failure makes it likely that no single agent will provide the long-desired cure. The likelihood is that we are entering the age of the 'critical care café' where patients will receive an individualized 'menu' of drugs and approaches that will work synergistically to improve their outcome. By then perhaps, various technologies will allow us to simultaneously assess epidemiological variables, demographic data, diagnoses, genetic predisposition, clinical phenotype, and many more variables to determine the appropriate therapeutic strategy for a specific patient. Sequential analysis of the patient's progression and continuous evaluation of response to therapies will guide the clinician in further tailoring therapy. Although this approach seems more like science-fiction than reality, this is the level of sophistication that will be required from the future ICUs and critical care physicians.

References

1. Zapol WM, Snider MT, Hill JD, et al (1979) Extracorporeal membrane oxygenation in severe acute respiratory failure. A randomized prospective study. JAMA 242:2193–2196
2. Abel SJ, Finney SJ, Brett SJ, Keogh BF, Morgan CJ, Evans TW (1998) Reduced mortality in association with the acute respiratory distress syndrome (ARDS). Thorax 53:292–294
3. Milberg JA, Davis DR, Steinberg KP, Hudson LD (1995) Improved survival of patients with acute respiratory distress syndrome (ARDS): 1983–1993. JAMA 273:306–309
4. Heyland DK, Cook DJ, Dodek PM (2002) Prevention of ventilator-associated pneumonia: Current practice in Canadian intensive care units. J Crit Care 17:161–167
5. Geerts W, Cook D, Selby R, Etchells E (2002) Venous thromboembolism and its prevention in critical care. J Crit Care 17:95–104
6. Cook D, Laporta D, Skrobik Y, et al (2001) Prevention of venous thromboembolism in critically ill surgery patients: a cross-sectional study. J Crit Care 16:161–166
7. The Acute Respiratory Distress Syndrome Network (2000) Ventilation with lower tidal volumes as compared with traditional tidal volumes for acute lung injury and the acute respiratory distress syndrome. N Engl J Med 342:1301–1308
8. Ayres SM, Grace WJ (1969) Inappropriate ventilation and hypoxemia as causes of cardiac arrhythmias. The control of arrhythmias without antiarrhythmic drugs. Am J Med 46:495–505
9. Argov Z, Mastaglia FL (1979) Drug therapy: Disorders of neuromuscular transmission caused by drugs. N Engl J Med 301:409–413
10. Le Bourdelles G, Viires N, Boczkowski J, Seta N, Pavlovic D, Aubier M (1994) Effects of mechanical ventilation on diaphragmatic contractile properties in rats. Am J Respir Crit Care Med 149:1539–1544
11. Petrof BJ, Legare M, Goldberg P, Milic-Emili J, Gottfried SB (1990) Continuous positive airway pressure reduces work of breathing and dyspnea during weaning from mechanical ventilation in severe chronic obstructive pulmonary disease. Am Rev Respir Dis 141:281–289
12. Sinderby C, Spahija J, Beck J (2001) Changes in respiratory effort sensation over time are linked to the frequency content of diaphragm electrical activity. Am J Respir Crit Care Med 163:905–910
13. Sinderby C, Navalesi P, Beck J, et al (1999) Neural control of mechanical ventilation in respiratory failure. Nat Med 5:1433–1436
14. Appendini L, Patessio A, Zanaboni S, et al (1994) Physiologic effects of positive end-expiratory pressure and mask pressure support during exacerbations of chronic obstructive pulmonary disease. Am J Respir Crit Care Med 149:1069–1076
15. Macklem PT (1984). Hyperinflation. Am Rev Respir Dis 129:1–2
16. Similowski T, Yan S, Gauthier AP, Macklem PT, Bellemare F (1991) Contractile properties of the human diaphragm during chronic hyperinflation. N Engl J Med 325:917–923
17. Ranieri VM, Giuliani R, Cinnella G, et al (1993) Physiologic effects of positive end-expiratory pressure in patients with chronic obstructive pulmonary disease during acute ventilatory failure and controlled mechanical ventilation. Am Rev Respir Dis 147:5–13
18. Sinderby CA, Beck JC, Lindstrom LH, Grassino AE (1997) Enhancement of signal quality in esophageal recordings of diaphragm EMG. J Appl Physiol 82:1370–1377

19. Beck J, Sinderby C, Lindstrom L, Grassino A (1998) Crural diaphragm activation during dynamic contractions at various inspiratory flow rates. J Appl Physiol 85:451–458
20. Sinderby CA, Beck JC, Lindstrom LH, Grassino AE (1997) Enhancement of signal quality in esophageal recordings of diaphragm EMG. J Appl Physiol 82:1370–1377
21. Beck J, Sinderby C, Lindstrom L, Grassino A (1996) Influence of bipolar esophageal electrode positioning on measurements of human crural diaphragm electromyogram. J Appl Physiol 81:1434–1449
22. Beck J, Sinderby C, Lindstrom L, Grassino A (1998) Effects of lung volume on diaphragm EMG signal strength during voluntary contractions. J Appl Physiol 85:1123–1134
23. Beck J, Sinderby C, Lindstrom L, Grassino A (1998) Effects of lung volume on diaphragm EMG signal strength during voluntary contractions. J Appl Physiol 85:1123–1134
24. Beck J, Gottfried SB, Navalesi P, et al (2001) Electrical activity of the diaphragm during pressure support ventilation in acute respiratory failure. Am J Respir Crit Care Med 164:419–424
25. Dreyfuss D, Saumon G (1998) Ventilator-induced lung injury: lessons from experimental studies. Am J Respir Crit Care Med 157:294–323
26. Slutsky AS (1999) Lung injury caused by mechanical ventilation. Chest 116 (Suppl):9S–15S
27. Tremblay LN, Slutsky AS (1998) Ventilator-induced injury: from barotrauma to biotrauma. Proc Assoc Am Physicians 110:482–488
28. Matamis D, Lemaire F, Harf A, Brun-Buisson C, Ansquer JC, Atlan G (1984) Total respiratory pressure-volume curves in the adult respiratory distress syndrome. Chest 86:58–66
29. Maggiore SM, Jonson B, Richard JC, Jaber S, Lemaire F, Brochard L (2001) Alveolar derecruitment at decremental positive end-expiratory pressure levels in acute lung injury: comparison with the lower inflection point, oxygenation, and compliance. Am J Respir Crit Care Med 164:795–801
30. Rimensberger PC, Cox PN, Frndova H, Bryan AC (1999) The open lung during small tidal volume ventilation: concepts of recruitment and "optimal" positive end-expiratory pressure. Crit Care Med 27:1946–1952
31. Ranieri VM, Grasso S, Mascia L, et al (1997) Effects of proportional assist ventilation on inspiratory muscle effort in patients with chronic obstructive pulmonary disease and acute respiratory failure. Anesthesiology 86:79–91
32. Brown BH, Barber DC, Seagar AD (1985) Applied potential tomography: possible clinical applications. Clin Phys Physiol Meas 6:109–121
33. Brown BH, Barber DC (1987) Electrical impedance tomography; the construction and application to physiological measurement of electrical impedance images. Med Prog Technol 13:69–75
34. Blott BH, Daniell GJ, Meeson S (1998) Electrical impedance tomography with compensation for electrode positioning variations. Phys Med Biol 43:1731–1739
35. Blott BH, Daniell GJ, Meeson S (1998) Nonlinear reconstruction constrained by image properties in electrical impedance tomography. Phys Med Biol 43:1215–1224
36. Kleinermann F, Avis NJ, Judah SK, Barber DC (1996) Three-dimensional image reconstruction for electrical impedance tomography. Physiol Meas 17 (Suppl 4A):A77–A83
37. Kunst PW, Vonk NA, Straver B, et al (1998) Influences of lung parenchyma density and thoracic fluid on ventilatory EIT measurements. Physiol Meas 19:27–34
38. Vonk NA, Kunst PW, Janse A, et al (1998) Pulmonary perfusion measured by means of electrical impedance tomography. Physiol Meas 19:263–273
39. Kunst PW, Vonk NA, Hoekstra OS, Postmus PE, de Vries PM (1998) Ventilation and perfusion imaging by electrical impedance tomography: a comparison with radionuclide scanning. Physiol Meas 19:481–490
40. Kunst PW, Vonk NA, Raaijmakers E, et al (1999) Electrical impedance tomography in the assessment of extravascular lung water in noncardiogenic acute respiratory failure. Chest 116:1695–1702

41. Frerichs I, Dudykevych T, Hinz J, Bodenstein M, Hahn G, Hellige G (2001) Gravity effects on regional lung ventilation determined by functional EIT during parabolic flights. J Appl Physiol 91:39–50
42. Frerichs I, Hahn G, Hellige G (1999) Thoracic electrical impedance tomographic measurements during volume controlled ventilation-effects of tidal volume and positive end-expiratory pressure. IEEE Trans Med Imaging 18:764–773
43. Frerichs I, Hahn G, Schroder T, Hellige G (1998) Electrical impedance tomography in monitoring experimental lung injury. Intensive Care Med 24:829–836
44. Frerichs I, Hahn G, Golisch W, Kurpitz M, Burchardi H, Hellige G (1998) Monitoring perioperative changes in distribution of pulmonary ventilation by functional electrical impedance tomography. Acta Anaesthesiol Scand 42:721–726
45. Kunst PW, Vazquez dA, Bohm SH, et al (2000) Monitoring of recruitment and derecruitment by electrical impedance tomography in a model of acute lung injury. Crit Care Med 28:3891–3895
46. Kunst PW, de Vries PM, Postmus PE, Bakker J (1999) Evaluation of electrical impedance tomography in the measurement of PEEP-induced changes in lung volume. Chest 115:1102–1106
47. Kunst PW, Bohm SH, Vazquez dA, et al (2000) Regional pressure volume curves by electrical impedance tomography in a model of acute lung injury. Crit Care Med 28:178–183
48. Eyuboglu BM, Brown BH, Barber DC (1988) Problems of cardiac output determination from electrical impedance tomography scans. Clin Phys Physiol Meas 9 (Suppl A):71–77
49. Eyuboglu BM, Brown BH, Barber DC, Seagar AD (1987) Localisation of cardiac related impedance changes in the thorax. Clin Phys Physiol Meas 8 (Suppl A):167–173
50. Leikauf GD, McDowell SA, Wesselkamper SC, et al (2002) Acute lung injury: functional genomics and genetic susceptibility. Chest 121 (3 Suppl):70S–75S
51. McDowell SA, Mallakin A, Bachurski CJ, et al (2002) The role of the receptor tyrosine kinase Ron in nickel-induced acute lung injury. Am J Respir Cell Mol Biol 26:99–104
52. Messer G, Spengler U, Jung MC, et al (1991) Polymorphic structure of the tumor necrosis factor (TNF) locus: an NcoI polymorphism in the first intron of the human TNF-beta gene correlates with a variant amino acid in position 26 and a reduced level of TNF-beta production. J Exp Med 173:209–219
53. Pociot F, Briant L, Jongeneel CV, et al (1993) Association of tumor necrosis factor (TNF) and class II major histocompatibility complex alleles with the secretion of TNF-alpha and TNF-beta by human mononuclear cells: a possible link to insulin-dependent diabetes mellitus. Eur J Immunol 23:224–231
54. Bouma G, Crusius JB, Oudkerk PM, et al (1996) Secretion of tumour necrosis factor alpha and lymphotoxin alpha in relation to polymorphisms in the TNF genes and HLA-DR alleles. Relevance for inflammatory bowel disease. Scand J Immunol 43:456–463
55. Stuber F, Petersen M, Bokelmann F, Schade U (1996) A genomic polymorphism within the tumor necrosis factor locus influences plasma tumor necrosis factor-alpha concentrations and outcome of patients with severe sepsis. Crit Care Med 24:381–384
56. Mira JP, Cariou A, Grall F, et al (1999) Association of TNF2, a TNF-alpha promoter polymorphism, with septic shock susceptibility and mortality: a multicenter study. JAMA 282:561–568
57. Stuber F, Udalova IA, Book M, et al (1995) -308 tumor necrosis factor (TNF) polymorphism is not associated with survival in severe sepsis and is unrelated to lipopolysaccharide inducibility of the human TNF promoter. J Inflamm 46:42–50
58. Waterer GW, Quasney MW, Cantor RM, Wunderink RG (2001) Septic shock and respiratory failure in community-acquired pneumonia have different TNF polymorphism associations. Am J Respir Crit Care Med 163:1599–1604
59. Majetschak M, Flohe S, Obertacke U, et al (1999) Relation of a TNF gene polymorphism to severe sepsis in trauma patients. Ann Surg 230:207–214

60. Marshall RP, Webb S, Bellingan GJ, et al (2002) Angiotensin converting enzyme insertion/deletion polymorphism is associated with susceptibility and outcome in acute respiratory distress syndrome. Am J Respir Crit Care Med 166:646–650
61. Baudin B (2002) New aspects on angiotensin-converting enzyme: from gene to disease. Clin Chem Lab Med 40:256–265
62. Vincent JL (2002) New management strategies in ARDS. Immunomodulation. Crit Care Clin 18:69–78
63. dos Santos CC, Chant C, Slutsky AS (2002) Pharmacotherapy of acute respiratory distress syndrome. Expert Opin Pharmacother 3:875–888
64. Ranieri VM, Suter PM, Tortorella C, et al (1999) Effect of mechanical ventilation on inflammatory mediators in patients with acute respiratory distress syndrome: a randomized controlled trial. JAMA 282:54–61
65. Ranieri VM, Giunta F, Suter PM, Slutsky AS (2000) Mechanical ventilation as a mediator of multisystem organ failure in acute respiratory distress syndrome. JAMA 284:43–44
66. Narimanbekov IO, Rozycki HJ (1995) Effect of IL-1 blockade on inflammatory manifestations of acute ventilator-induced lung injury in a rabbit model. Exp Lung Res 21:239–254
67. Ulich TR, Yin SM, Guo KZ, del Castillo J, Eisenberg SP, Thompson RC (1991) The intratracheal administration of endotoxin and cytokines. III. The interleukin-1 (IL-1) receptor antagonist inhibits endotoxin- and IL-1-induced acute inflammation. Am J Pathol 138:521–524
68. Leff JA, Bodman ME, Cho OJ, et al (1994) Post-insult treatment with interleukin-1 receptor antagonist decreases oxidative lung injury in rats given intratracheal interleukin-1. Am J Respir Crit Care Med 150:109–112
69. Imai Y, Kawano T, Iwamoto S, Nakagawa S, Takata M, Miyasaka K (1999) Intratracheal anti-tumor necrosis factor-alpha antibody attenuates ventilator-induced lung injury in rabbits. J Appl Physiol 87:510–515
70. Shvedova AA, Kramarik JA, Keohavong P, Chumakov KM, Karol MH (1994) Use of anti-TNF-alpha antiserum to investigate toxic alveolitis arising from cotton dust exposure. Exp Lung Res 20:297–315
71. Weiss YG, Maloyan A, Tazelaar J, Raj N, Deutschman CS (2002) Adenoviral transfer of HSP-70 into pulmonary epithelium ameliorates experimental acute respiratory distress syndrome. J Clin Invest 110:801–806
72. Asea A, Kabingu E, Stevenson MA, Calderwood SK (2000) HSP70 peptidembearing and peptide-negative preparations act as chaperokines. Cell Stress Chaperones 5:425–431
73. Asea A, Kraeft SK, Kurt-Jones EA, et al (2000) HSP70 stimulates cytokine production through a CD14-dependant pathway, demonstrating its dual role as a chaperone and cytokine. Nat Med 6:435–442
74. Xie Y, Cahill CM, Asea A, Auron PE, Calderwood SK (1999) Heat shock proteins and regulation of cytokine expression. Infect Dis Obstet Gynecol 7:26–30
75. Asea A, Rehli M, Kabingu E, et al (2002) Novel signal transduction pathway utilized by extracellular HSP70: role of toll-like receptor (TLR) 2 and TLR4. J Biol Chem 277:15028–15034
76. Vabulas RM, Ahmad-Nejad P, Ghose S, Kirschning CJ, Issels RD, Wagner H (2002) HSP70 as endogenous stimulus of the Toll/interleukin-1 receptor signal pathway. J Biol Chem 277:15107–15112
77. Frerichs I, Schiffmann H, Hahn G, Hellige G (2001) Non-invasive radiation-free monitoring of regional lung ventilation in critically ill infants. Intensive Care Med 27:1385–139410.
78. Frerichs I, Hinz J, Herrmann P, et al (2002) Detection of local lung air content by electrical impedance tomography compared with electron beam CT. J Appl Physiol 93:660–666

Subject Index

A
acute
- exacerbations 79
- - of COPD 90
- - prevention 90
- lung injury (ALI) 23, 67, 68, 74, 143, 149
- myocardial infarction 56
- respiratory distress syndrome (ARDS) 5, 8, 15, 21, 67, 74, 144, 155
- respiratory failure 32, 149
- severe asthma 62
- tracheobronchitis 88, 89
agitation 135
airflow resistance 29
airway injury 130
alcohol 114
alcohol-based
- solution 112
- antiseptics 111
- gel 112
alcoholic solution 110
ALI, see acute lung injury
alveolar
- collapse 143
- derecruitment 23
- recruitment 14, 67
ALVECLI 144
- trial 76
aminoglycosides 141
aminopenicillins 88
amoxicillin 85, 88, 89
ampicillin 86, 87
angiotensin (AT) 159
- angiotensin converting enzyme (ACE) gene
- - D allele 159
anticholinergic agent 82
antiseptic products 117
anti-TNF-α antibody (Ab) 161
anxiety 135
APACHE III score 126

ARDS (see also acute respiratory distress syndrome) 5, 8, 15, 25, 68, 149
- extrapulmonary 22
- pulmonary 22
ARDS Network 144, 160
aspiration 129
assist-control mode 7
atelectrauma 155
atracuronium 140
auto-PEEP 150
axonal change 135

B
BAL (bronchoalveolar lavage) 101, 104, 158
barotrauma 150, 155
beta-agonist
- long-acting 82
- short-acting 82
biotrauma 155, 159
blinded bronchial sampling (BBS) 103
blood cultures 150
Bordetella pertussis 88
bradykinin 159
bronchoalveolar lavage (BAL) 101, 104, 158

C
cardiogenic pulmonary edema 56, 57
case-control 42
cefixime 88
cefprozil 88
cefuroxine 88
cephalosporins 87, 88
CESAR trial 146
Chlamydia pneumoniae 88
chloramphenicol 86
chlorhexidine 114
chronic
- bronchitis 89
- - acute exacerbation 80

- obstructive pulmonary disease (COPD)   5, 14, 121, 150
- - acute exacerbation   79
- respiratory failure   51
Ciaglia technique   131, 133
cigarette smoking   90
CINAHL   74
ciprofloxacin   88, 89
clavulanate   85, 88
CO_2
- extracorporeal removal   16
co-amoxiclav   86
Cochrane Controlled Trials Register   74, 122
Cochrane Data Base of Systematic Reviews   74, 122, 143
coma   123, 129
community-acquired pneumonia   21
compliance   31, 34
- total   31
continuous positive airway pressure (CPAP)   56, 70
COPD   41
- exacerbation   54, 55
corticosteroids   85, 141, 146
cotrimoxazole   86
cuff leak   41
Cumulative Index to Nursing and Allied Health Literature (CINAHL)   122

D
daily SBT   40
decelerating flow   14
deep vein thrombosis (DVT)   45, 149
derecruitment   34, 69
diaphragm   150, 152, 155
Doppler ultrasound   46
doxycycline   86, 88, 89
duplex ultrasound   48

E
electrical impedance tomography   155
EMBASE   74, 143
emergency ward   55
endothelial cell-leukocyte adhesion molecule-1 (ELAM-1)   162
endotracheal aspirates   101, 104
- qualitative   105
enkephalins   159
erythromycin   87
EXPRESS   144
extracorporeal membrane oxygenation (ECMO)   16, 146
extravascular lung water   157

extubation   41

F
FACCT trial   146
fiberoptic bronchoscopy   102
fluid management   146
fluoroquinolones   88
forced expiratory value in one second (FEV_1)   81
frequency/tidal volume ratio (f/V_T)   39
full face mask   41
functional residual capacity   31

G
gram-negative
- bacilli   109
- culture   115
Griggs technique   133

H
Haemophilus
- influenzae   88, 89
- spp.   89
hand hygiene   109, 113, 116, 117
handrubbing   113
handwashing   110, 112114
HealthSTAR   74
heat shock protein   161
helium-oxygen mixture   56
hydrocortisone   83
hypoxemic respiratory failure   58
immunomodulation   160
immunosuppression   61
infection rates   114
inflection point
- lower   31, 67
- upper   31
influenza   91
- A   91
- B   91
- vaccination   91
inhaled
- nitric oxide   74, 145
- steroids   84
intrinsic positive end-expiratory pressure (PEEPi)   21, 127
intubation   55
- reduction   55
iodinated glycerol   91

K
Klebsiella   113, 116
- spp.   89

L

β-lactam
- antibiotics 87
- inhibitor 87

β-lactamase
- inhibitor 87
- producing bacteria 87

Late Steroid Rescue Study 146
leukotrine (LT) receptor antagonists 90
likelihood ratios 39
Literatura Latino Americana y del Caribe de Información en Ciencias de la Salud (LILACS) 122
lung
- function (FEV$_1$) 81, 88
- protective strategy 23, 74
- surgery 61

Lung Open Ventilation Study 144

M

M. catarrhalis 88, 89
macrolides 87, 88
maximum inspiratory pressure 39
MEDLINE 74, 122, 143
methicillin-resistant S. aureus (MRSA) 115, 116
methylprednisolone 83, 85
methylxanthines 82
microarray analyses 158
midazolam 136138
molecular genetics 158
monitoring 29
mortality 9, 15
mucolytic agents 91
Mycoplasma pneumoniae 88
myopathic change 135

N

N-acetylcysteine 91, 92
neurally adjusted ventilatory assist (NAVA) 150
neuramidase inhibitors 91
neuromuscular
- blocker 135, 141
- disease 121, 123, 129
- junction 155

neurosurgical patients 47
neurotensin 159
neutrophil elastase inhibitor 147
nitric oxide 160
non-elastic forces 29
non-invasive ventilation (NIV) 90
nosocomial pneumonia 126, 129

nuclear factor-kappa B 162

O

ofloxacin 86
overdistention 21
overstretching 21, 22
oxytetracycline 86

P

pancuronium 137, 140
PCV 23
PDT, see percutaneous dilatational tracheostomy
- endoscopically guided 128

peak
- expiratory flow rates 81
- inspiratory pressure 14

PEEP, see positive end-expiratory pressure
penicillin resistance 87
percutaneous dilatational tracheostomy (PDT) 128, 132
perioperative bleeding 132
phrenic nerve 15
plateau pressure 21
pneumococcal vaccination 91
pneumonia 8, 41
positive end-expiratory pressure (PEEP) 8, 22, 32, 37, 67, 68, 76, 144
- auto-PEEP 150

post-extubation respiratory failure 61
post-hoc analysis 39
prednisone 83, 85
pressure
- maximum inspiratory 39
- peak inspiratory 14
- plateau pressure 21
- pressure/volume (P/V) 67
- - curve 76, 155
- support (PS) 7, 13
- - plus PEEP 56
- transpulmonary 24
- volume (P/V) loop 31

progressive withdrawal 40
prone
- position 23
- ventilation 144

prophylaxis 47
propofol 136138
protected specimen brush samples (PSB) 102, 104
Pseudomonas aeruginosa 88, 89
PSV 39, 41
pulmonary

- arterial catheter 146
- embolism 45
- mechanics 29, 30, 127

R
Ramsay 137, 139
randomized controlled trial 21, 22, 39
reabsorption atelectasis 22
receptor tyrosine kinase Ron 158
recombinant
- human atrial natriuretic peptide 147
- IL-1 receptor antagonist (IL-1ra) 160
recruitment maneuver 24, 67, 68
reintubation 41, 123, 126, 129
renal failure 141
respiratory center 150, 155

S
sedation 135
- algorithm 141
sedative blocker 135
sigh 70
SIMV 7, 41
single daily trial 40
smoking cessation 90
soap
- antiseptic 112
- medicated 111
- nonmediated 111, 114
spontaneous breathing 39
sputum gram stain 81
Staphylococcus aureus 109
Streptococcus pneumoniae 87, 89
substance P 159
sulphamethoxazole 87, 89

T
tetracycline 8688
therapy
- aerosol 129
- antibiotic 84
- antimicrobial 88
- bronchodilator 82
- corticosteroids 83
- surfactant 146
tidal volume 7, 21, 25, 31, 143
- limitation 74, 75
T-piece 39, 40
tracheostomy 121, 123, 126130
- non-surgical 128
- percutaneous dilatational 128, 131
- percutaneous non-surgical 127
- surgical 127, 128, 131133

- translaryngeal 131, 133
translaryngeal intubation 130
transpulmonary pressure 24
triclosan 115
trimethaprim-sulphamethoxazole 88
trimethoprim 87, 89
tumor necrosis factor (TNF)
- α-308 gene polymorphism 159
- β gene 159
- receptor associated factor 162

U
ultrasonography 47
unfractionated heparin 47
upper airway obstruction 41

V
V/Q ratio 24
vancomycin-resistant enterococci (VRE) 116
vecuronium 137, 140
venography 46
venous thromboembolism 45
ventilation
- alveolar 25
- dead space 127
- high frequency 14
- - oscillatory 15
- - vs. conventional 15
- intermittent mandatory 131
- low frequency 16
- lung-protective 73
- mechanical 6, 67, 123
- neural control 149
- non-invasive 41
- - mechanical 7
- open lung 74, 76, 143
- partial liquid 160
- pressure controlled 14, 15
- pressure-controlled 23
- synchronized intermittent mandatory (SIMV) 13
- volume controlled 15, 68
ventilation-perfusion
- ratio 23
- scans 45
ventilator
- disconnection 69
- modes 13
- settings 7
ventilator-associated pneumonia (VAP) 99, 149
ventilator-induced injury 22
ventilogenomics 158, 160

volume control mode 7, 14
volutrauma 155
VRE 116

W

weaning 37, 121, 127, 130, 131, 135
– failure 40
– predictors 37, 39, 41
– protocols 42
– success 39
work of breathing (WOB) 14, 40, 127, 131